G000253148

LYDIA CAMPBELL'S
ULTIMATE
Legs Bums 'N' Tums

BOXTREE

Advice to the Reader

Before following any medical or dietary advice contained in this book, it is recommended that you consult your doctor if you suffer from any health problems or special conditions or are in any doubt as to its suitability.

First published in Great Britain in 1996 by
Boxtree Limited, Broadwall House, 21 Broadwall, London
SE1 9PL

Copyright © Lydia Campbell 1996

The right of Lydia Campbell to be identified as Author of this work has been asserted by her in accordance with the Copyright, Designs and Patents Act 1988

All rights reserved

1 3 5 7 9 10 8 6 4 2

ISBN 0 7522 0556 0

Designed by **DW Design**
Cover designed by **Slatter~Anderson**
Photographs © **Damian Walker**

Except in the United States of America this book is sold subject to the condition that it shall not, by way of trade or otherwise, be lent, resold, hired out or otherwise circulated without the publisher's prior consent in any form of binding or cover other than that in which it is published and without a similar condition including this condition being imposed upon a subsequent purchaser.

Printed and bound in Great Britain by Butler & Tanner

A CIP catalogue entry for this book is available from the British Library

Acknowledgements

To my husband and work colleague Steve Evans, to my daughters Rayne, Hester, Sara and Antonia, and to my mother all of whose unconditional love has been my source of inspiration, determination and achievement.

To Laura Connell and my manager Vicki McIvor for helping me see the project through.

To my team of International FitCamp presenters who have honoured my work and beliefs for so many years.

To Vicky Monk, Sarah Bennie and all at Boxtree for their help and enthusiasm.

To all those men and women who are searching to find their real selves.

To all the thousands of students and teachers who have been to my events, work-outs and studio.
Thank you for your energy, support and feedback.

Contents

Welcome to the *Ultimate Legs Bums 'N' Tums programme*. In the early Eighties, I created the first Legs Bums 'N' Tums class to complement the aerobics classes I was running in my original fitness studio, Stripes, in Ealing, London, which measured 35ft by 27ft. Within three months of opening, the studio had 3,000 members.

It was the Jane Fonda boom time. As studio manager, I was a unique role model. I was not a hard-bodied, 21-year-old aerobics teacher, I was a fit young mother of three. Because of this, I attracted all shapes, sizes and ages to my classes. I had to cater for all levels of fitness.

Legs Bums 'N' Tums (LBT) was created for women to focus on muscle, for those women who were put off by the no-pain, no-gain aerobic attitude that one would encounter in a typical aerobic class.

What started out as an alternative class on my timetable has grown into one of the most popular work-outs throughout the nation.

After a few years of teaching LBT I felt there was something missing. Women were asking me to monitor their progress, to weigh them and to give nutritional advice. This happened soon after the birth of my fourth daughter.

Personally, I was having a battle with my own body shape and body image yet I was fit, in shape and teaching six to eight classes a week. I developed the Ultimate Legs, Bums 'N' Tums (ULBT) programme to look at lifestyle, activity levels, eating habits and body image. Studio members could join in the networking session linked to the class afterwards where all these issues were addressed and a personal monitoring system created to address them.

As a result of these sessions, I saw results in women who had always battled with their weight and self-esteem. These women were taking responsibility for the long-term success of reaching their inward and outward goals. They weren't simply coming to class expecting to be transformed anymore. They learned about themselves and what it takes to achieve their goals.

It has taken me a long time to write this book. Here it is, finally, after years of personal experience, research, teaching and talking to hundreds of people, all who inspired me to get my message out there. I would like to thank you because if it were not for you I would not have done this.

My main message is that it is time to stop being conned and take responsibility for yourself, your shape, your health, your eating and lifestyle. Once you understand what you can realistically achieve through the programme you can accept a realistic new you and you will never have a weight problem, or look at a diet book again.

Welcome to the ULBT programme – get ready for change!

Why you failed

Most diet books are centred around calorie-counting, cooking and low-fat meal planning, claiming that this will be the answer to transforming your shape short term, maybe for life. Some do emphasize the importance of exercise, but the fact is that there has been an imbalance of accurate information. Weight has always been the issue. Dieting is still seen as the answer to the new you. More people attend diet clubs than exercise clubs in the UK and USA. More money is spent on diet aids or gimmicks than is spent on becoming healthy and I am talking about millions of pounds. One of the main reasons why I have written this book is because having been in the fitness and health business since the late Seventies, I have seen all the trends and the diet fads. In my twenties I must have tried every diet possible in search of a beautiful physique - from brown rice diets to complete fasting. However, when I became the studio manager of one of the first multi-functional health clubs in London, exercise was all I believed in.

As a fitness professional, I frowned upon the slimming world. What actually happened was that people decided either to take up exercise by joining the aerobic classes, or to try every diet out there and go for weigh-ins at slimming clubs. Then the situation became worse. The combination of fad diets and extreme exercising filtered into the fitness world and everyone, from instructors to celebrities, were exercising three to four hours a day and living off next to nothing. This occurred in the late Eighties. In 1995, Jane Fonda finally admitted to the unreality of this lifestyle.

Meanwhile, from the mid-Eighties well into the Nineties, eating disorders became the norm and exercise fanatics sought their fix everyday with long gruelling work-outs. While the slimming world has come to terms with the fact that the public cannot be tricked into dieting anymore and now promote healthy eating plans, there are still so many confused messages. It is no wonder that people give up or do not even attempt to lead a healthier lifestyle. This is what the ULBT programme is all about. It is based on the exercise format, which I created and developed in the early Eighties, for women to achieve realistic goals by combining healthy eating with regular exercise. I now share it with you.

The programme sounds very simple, but I go into depth to address the reasons why you may be hooked on dieting and what you can do to change; why your body image plays such an important role on your decisions regarding food choices, exercise and lifestyle; and the exercise programme is included – a programme where you take the responsibility for making a commitment to shaping up. There are masses of exercises to choose from for variety and staying power.

If you are new to exercise, it is going to take time for you to work through the programme. If you are more experienced you may need the added benefits of using resistance equipment to challenge your body.

There is a chapter on aerobics because aerobics has always been part of my LBT class. You can't use up body fat any other way except through regular aerobic work-outs. This does not mean you have to do aerobic dance. I am talking about all forms of fat-burning exercise which you will read about in Chapter 7.

Before you start the programme, I am going to address the issue of failure and why the diet programme has failed you.

Where did you go wrong before?

Maybe you have tried numerous diet and exercise programmes which have failed you. Was it because your expectations were too high? Did the diet or exercise claim you would transform yourself in ten to twenty-one days? The days of claims are over and marketing and advertising campaigns need to wise-up to the fact that the public can't be tricked anymore into thinking that a programme or diet will transform you into the shape of the supermodel used as the promoter.

I'm being honest with you. Your failure is due to unrealistic expectations. At the end of the day real results take time, patience and hard work. You have to make the decision to be responsible for the way you eat and exercise – not for a few weeks but for life.

When you start an exercise programme or diet and look at a height-and-weight chart do you say to yourself, 'I'm going to lose two stone', or do you see that you do not meet the weight stated, that in fact you are way above average in weight for your height and so you feel obese because that is what the chart is showing you? What is your ideal weight you may wonder?

How much should you weigh?

This is not easy to answer as height-and-weight tables give you an acceptable range. Most are outdated and none have been designed from statistics based on fit people. Fit people usually weigh more than the chart's acceptable range because muscle weighs more than fat.

The true measure should be based on body fat, which a chart or weighing scales cannot detect on an individual. Ideally, a man's body – fat level should be 15–20 percent of the body mass and woman's between 20–25 percent. It is the amount of lean body mass compared to the amount of body fat that really counts.

You may want to have a fitness professional measure your body fat but be warned, the only accurate method is hydrostatic weighing which is done in water under laboratory conditions.

Should you weigh yourself?

Stepping on scales is, for most people, totally misleading as your body weight fluctuates throughout the day. Scales can also differ. Remember that they cannot account for one's body composition.

As you get fitter following the programme, you may find that your weight does not change because muscle weight replaces fat weight. It may even increase, but you will find that your clothing size becomes smaller.

The aim is to improve one's lean muscle mass. The more muscle you have compared to body fat, the more calories you will burn in your everyday living. Do not be frightened of having muscle – it only means your body will have a firm, toned shape. Your body won't wobble when you walk, run or dance – except for your bust!

Having muscle does not mean looking like a sculpted body-builder. This is an extreme look achieved by hours of hard training and by maintaining an unhealthy low body fat from excessive dieting – not recommended for the average body.

Most women cannot develop enormous bulky muscle because our hormones restrict this type of muscle growth. It is the male hormone testosterone that increases muscle growth. We all have male and female hormones. Some women can develop far more muscle naturally than others because they have a naturally higher testosterone level than others. Muscle size is also related to your genetic make-up.

How can you change your level of body fat?

You can only decrease your body fat level by the combination of regular aerobic exercise and low-fat healthy eating. You need to exercise aerobically for twenty to thirty minutes, four to five times a week for fat loss, plus three to four sessions a week of muscular-strength training. This is what the ULBT programme is all about.

You may have tried every diet but you still have not become the shape you expected. Maybe you lost weight from your bust and not the desired inches from your hips. Why?

The answer is to understand your body shape.

Your body shape

Before we were born our basic body shape was determined by our genes. Our genetic make-up is inherited from our parents and grandparents and it dictates our shape, colouring and features. Our actual shape is based on three body types.

Mesomorph (think of Madonna) = muscular, a natural athletic build, large-boned, wide shoulders, no real waist, narrow hips. Mesomorphs can store fat around the torso and legs.

Endomorph (think of Cindy Crawford) = round, curvy, wide hips, often with smaller upper bodies. Endomorphs have a tendency to store a high percentage of fat.

Ectomorph (think of Claudia Schiffer) = slender, long-limbed build, not much muscle. Ectomorphs do not usually have a weight problem.

Very few of us are one shape. Most are a mix. I'm a meso-endomorph. All I have to do is blink and I have a muscle, but I'm short and chunky with curves and a tendency to store fat around my middle and thighs. I inherited my father's wide shoulders and ribs and my mother's backside and thighs - a perfect build for power and explosive work.

As a child, I excelled in most sports and dance. My dream was to be a professional ballet dancer. In those days, you were measured and weighed at a certain stage. The effect on my body image was a nightmare. After ten years of classical ballet, I left heartbroken when I was informed I would not make the grade. I was expected to be too tall as I had large bones, weighed too much and had size seven feet. For some reason, I never grew past 5ft 4ins. I blame it on my genes.

So, have a good look at the builds in your family. Observe who has the height. What build are they? Who has long limbs? Who has stocky, muscular limbs? Who do you take after?

Watching four daughters growing up is fascinating because while they all had similar birth weights and were brought up on the same diet, they are all different in build. One is tall and meso-endomorphic, one is very mesomorphic, one is pear-shaped and predominantly endomorphic. The youngest looks very ectomorphic but it is too early to tell her shape for certain.

Whatever shape you are, you want to be the best you can realistically achieve based on your genetic make-up. You won't develop broad, muscular shoulders if you are genetically an ectomorph, or have long, slender limbs if you are a powerful short mesomorph. It is vital to realize that a well-shaped body that's firm, not fat, doesn't necessarily mean small, thin, petite or slender.

One main reason why diets do not work is because most slimming diets are not scientifically based. Most diets do not deal with the issue of healthy eating. Following a faddy diet or an extreme low-calorie diet can be quite dangerous for your health. With the ULBT programme I do not state that you should eat a restrictive low-calorie diet because I am not a dietician, but I do advocate the National

Food Guide information which addresses the problem of how to plan and enjoy healthy eating.

You may have tried magic diet aids from pills and wraps to potions, but the only thing that is permanently thinner is your purse. The effects of crash dieting, slimming foods, drinks and meal replacement bars is short-lived. It is mainly water and lean body tissue that is lost, not fat. Once you return to normal eating there is an immediate weight gain. So you diet again and you enter the yo-yo diet syndrome. People who do this have a tendency to put on more weight every time they resume their normal eating pattern.

I am only discussing briefly the issue of weight loss since to succeed with the ULBT programme you have to forget scales and drastic calorie cutting. You are entering a reality programme to enable you to reach your goals permanently.

If you are very overweight your muscles are slack and your body is flabby. It is going to take a great deal of time to tone and firm those muscles. Do not expect results overnight. Whatever you've read before, you cannot achieve a new toned you in nine, fifteen or twenty hours or days. It is impossible for the body to drop excess fat in such a short time. Any rapid weight loss in the first couple of weeks is predominately water weight. Do not despair at these words because the more you understand now, the more you will be able to achieve and control later. Finally, everyone responds differently to diet and exercise. No two people have the same results. If you understand this, you may stop competing and being influenced by friends or by diet claims.

What it takes to get results

The hardest part of any programme or form of regular exercise is to simply get up off the couch and move that body. You do want to do it, otherwise you would not be reading this book. Of course there are other reasons, maybe one of the following is yours:

1. Curiosity. What is the ULBT programme about?
2. You want to shape up for a special occasion.
3. You want to change your shape permanently.
4. You are already into exercise yet you are always looking for new ways and new exercises to keep yourself in shape.
5. You have never exercised before, except during your school days and now you feel it is time to lead a healthier lifestyle.
6. You have been told for medical reasons that you have to get yourself into shape.
7. You are a mother and you want to shift the excess flab and tone your tum.
8. Maybe you are always working and have never made time to work-out. You are looking for a programme that can fit into your timetable.

Whatever your reason, I want the ULBT programme to work for you. My aim is to help you make permanent lifestyle changes to get and maintain results that will, in turn, help you to achieve your personal goals.

There have been numerous exercise books, systems and exercise experts all claiming that if you follow a particular method you will be transformed, especially within a short period of time. Maybe you have tried the softer options of pills, slimming potions, drinks, body wraps and massage machines to achieve a loss of inches, spending a fortune on gimmicks that do not work long-term. Some only last for a matter of a few hours until you drink back the fluid that has been squeezed and extracted from your body. Maybe you have continually dieted, trying out every possible diet to shift the flab. You have lost weight and then lost control and it has all piled back

on – and more. The truth is that none of it works. All the latest research is coming up with the same answers. The only way to lose weight permanently is by combining an effective regular exercise programme with sound nutritional eating habits in a combination that you can follow for life. The ULBT programme consists of making lifestyle changes. It creates nutritional awareness and offers effective body–shaping exercises, from aerobic training to spot training for all those problem areas.

It is mainly for vanity reasons that most people choose to diet and exercise. Very few start any diet or exercise programme for health reasons unless instructed by their doctor.

I want the ULBT programme to work for you to firm the flab, but I also hope the programme will re-educate your attitude toward dieting and exercise. You will learn to make permanent lifestyle changes to get and maintain results. Do not worry, this does not mean you are on a diet for life, that is the last thing I want you to think. Diets are out as far as I am concerned, you will learn about this later.

The drop-out factor

To begin with, I'm going to address the issue of becoming active and staying active. This is because so many of your good intentions about achieving results disappear into thin air within a few months and you simply drop out. It is the drop-out factor that seems to rule most of us. If you are mentally prepared beforehand for all the emotional and practical hurdles that get in the way of achieving results, you'll get over them, face your problems, tackle them and carry on. So let's get started.

The majority of us who start an exercise programme drop out within six months. If you can get past six months, you will find yourself committed to exercise. By that time it is in your blood and you would miss it if you could not work-out. You may think you could never reach this feeling because you have always been an exercise drop-out. My aim is for you to become self-motivated and disciplined, and to be able to stick to the programme. So why does it happen to you? Why can you not stick to a programme? What are the hurdles that blocked you?

I have no time to work-out.

This is the biggest excuse – life always take you over. This is where self-discipline comes in. Switch off from the demands of life around you. Every day set aside time to exercise, even if it is only ten minutes. If you have time to watch TV, you have time to exercise. Once you know the exercises, you can even do them while watching TV. Make an appointment with yourself and stick to it. If you are a workaholic, justify the exercise time by using it for creative thinking. Give yourself the mental space to walk away from the office and workload to focus on yourself.

The good news is that even short sessions of exercise work for you. Research from the American College of Sports Medicine and USA Centers for Disease Control has shown that if your life is predominately sedentary and you take the steps to accumulate thirty minutes of moderate exercise on most days, you will achieve a substantial reduction in your risk of heart disease and certain forms of cancer. Health issues may not be so important to you, vanity is the main reason we work-out. But let's be honest, why do you not want the added benefits of getting more out of life by being healthier?

I know all too well how you feel when you have no time to work-out. My life is always hectic. Rarely do I have a smooth-running day, so much goes on that a day can feel like a week and a week in my life can be so frantic that I cannot remember how it started. Time is extremely precious to me.

I used to be so hard on myself about housework standards and mess. This is one priority I've dropped with an active family of six. The house is usually in chaos, because we are not perfect. The laundry area looks like a bomb site! I am forever rummaging through piles of clothes looking for knickers or a favourite leotard. It sounds peculiar, but relaxing certain standards gives you more quality time in life to be productive, creative, have fun and de-stress.

Time is precious and cannot be replaced. It is time you took a step back and let something go. If you prioritize what is really important to you, allowing ten minutes a day for exercise, you'll get more out of the other twenty-three hours and fifty minutes.

I never have the energy to work-out and I am always tired.

Mentally you feel sluggish at the end of a day. You have thoughts that sway you away from exercise. The moment you make the decision to change, your subconscious creates barriers because you are simply too tired. You always seem to end the day with the thought that tomorrow is a new day, exercise can begin then. The mind will always try to turn a positive thought into a negative. Learn to use mental muscle, do not get distracted. Stay focused on the programme and exercise, you will then achieve the instant pay-off of feeling good, re-energized and ready for anything.

I never feel like exercising.

Create the energy, change your negative feelings by simply going for it. Fresh air is an energy stimulant. If you have been stuck in a stuffy, hot work environment all day of course you will feel tired. Re-energize with a brisk walk around the block before you step indoors. Walk fast, breathe deeply and focus on the exercise session to come. Exercise the moment you get into the house. Simply change your clothes and work-out – even if you are talking about the day to family, flatmates or friends – work-out as you do it – it is a great way of releasing stress.

I am absolutely hopeless in the evening, all I want to do is sleep.

You may be one of those people who wake up with the dawn and can simply jump out of bed totally refreshed needing no caffeine fix to stimulate your thoughts for the day. I fall into this category, daylight and a good sleep gives me energy; in the summer I am almost an insomniac. The morning is the best time of the day for my personal work-out, maybe it is the best time for you – try it. Your tiredness and sluggish feeling may be due to your diet. What you eat twenty-four hours earlier affects your energy levels. Read Chapter 4 and make food choice changes to fuel your body. Soon you will have the energy to tackle anything.

I am sleepy during the day and at the end of the day I am positively knackered.

Your diet plays an important role here but another aid is power napping – the American term for a quick snooze or cat-nap. Take a power nap in your lunch time, or if you are at home try a mid-afternoon siesta. Twenty minutes of sleep can give you an enormous energy boost.

Finally on tiredness, the mind will always create negative thoughts, blocking you from being active, you simply have to go for it, even if it is only doing the ten-minute work-out to start with. You will create an energy boost while exercising. Exercise is strange, most people never feel like it but once they have worked-out they feel great. It is the feel-good factor that keeps you energized.

I started a programme but it was too hard, it hurt, I could not take the pace and dropped out.

Do not go mad when you are new to exercise. Take it one step at a time. Work-out at the level that is suitable for you as stated in the exercise programme. Often the feel-good factor takes over while exercising and doing too much too soon creates extreme muscle soreness and sometimes injury.

Learn how to monitor your work-out intensity, duration and frequency. The three most simple self-monitoring methods are the talk test, listening to your body and feeling pain.

The talk test: can you talk comfortably while you are exercising? This doesn't mean gasping a few words, it means being able to hold a conversation and breathing deeply at the same time.

Listening to your body: is the pace too easy or too hard? As you talk to yourself while exercising, focus on how you feel. Is the pace leaving you breathless (too fast) or can you recite a poem (too slow)? Find a comfortable pace which you can sustain for a twenty-to-thirty minute work-out.

Pain. Is it painful? Are you going for the burn?: do not work-out at a level at which you feel the burn during the aerobic sessions. Feeling the burn means that the waste products created by the muscle effort are building up – you are working out too hard, beyond an aerobic training range. You are now in an anaerobic mode when your muscles require no oxygen for movement. Short bursts of high energy moves are anaerobic. For calorie burning, you don't want this to happen. Slow down and pace yourself so that you feel comfortable. There should be no muscle burning, and you should be able to continue this pace for twenty to thirty minutes.

The easiest way of monitoring how hard an intensity should be is by using a target heart-rate range chart and by pulse taking. You need to work-out at the training range appropriate for your age and fitness level.

A beginner should work-out to 60 percent of their training range, those more advanced up to 85 percent (page 70).

If you can afford it, invest in a heart-rate monitor such as a Polar Heart Rate Monitor; a fascinating and most effective training tool. Your heart rate is the most important factor in effective weight loss and heart health (cardiovascular fitness). A heart-rate monitor is the most accurate method of monitoring your work-out intensity. Too low a heart rate and you will not be on a training level, you will gain no results and no benefit. Training at too high a rate means that you are making your heart work too hard, you are uncomfortable and you cannot keep up the pace. Too high a training level can lead to injury, pain and extreme fatigue.

During your safe training range, your heart rate is working at a comfortable level without unnecessary strain. This level is the only effective way to burn calories, body fat and increase your level of aerobic fitness. Using a monitor such as a Polar Monitor makes it so simple to know how hard you are working. You don't have to be an athlete to use one. I would recommend you get one especially as self-monitoring by pulse taking is not really accurate.

Duration. For how long should I exercise?

Time will actually fly by when you exercise, as your thoughts focus on your work-out. Beginners should aim for ten to fifteen minutes. If this is too easy, progress to twenty to thirty minutes, then progress to thirty minutes. Those used to exercising should work-out for a minimum of twenty to thirty minutes.

If you want to burn up excess calories and fat, the key is to be able to exercise for twenty to thirty minutes per session. As your fitness level improves with time, you will be able to work-out for thirty-minute sessions and burn more calories. The longer you exercise, the better. For a beginner this may mean long brisk walks for aerobic training. If I said you had to run a mile you would not get far, the intensity and duration of the exercise would be too much. As you get fitter, running a mile will become no problem.

Frequency. How often should I work-out?

Following the programme once a week is a total waste of time, the only benefit will be mental release. You will only get physical results if you exercise a minimum of three to four times a week, for a period of twenty to thirty minutes at a training intensity for

you. Because you are aiming to use up calories as you train, this will not happen if you are working-out at a leisurely walking pace.

I became demotivated – it was boring and tedious.

Firstly, I have already spoken about training levels and you now know that exercising at too hard a level too intensely will lead to pain and sometimes injury. Pain is a huge demotivator – it is not motivating when it hurts. If exercise is not fun you will get bored and simply stop. Exercising at home is extremely hard anyway. Self-discipline and commitment to yourself is the key. I cannot come and personally train you, I can only try and inspire you to stick at it via this book.

The following are my own personal self-motivation tips:

* Carry or place in a prominent position the worst picture of yourself. A fleeting glance at this photo will remind you of what you do not want to look like. I have numerous choices! Pictures of me are in my purse, another in my bedside drawer, another in my desk drawer – pictures of me not at my best when I was inactive after I had a knee accident and was desk-bound due to my workload. The weight piled on. I was depressed at the time and overeating due to stress. This sounds like a very negative approach, but I assure you it motivates you not to return to that state!

* Go to the other extreme – prominently display a poster of a body you love. I love pictures of well-defined men. The sexiness and sleekness of their muscles is enough for me to say, 'Yes, I will work at my body'. You may be inspired by a woman's shape. Whatever your inspiration, stick up a few posters where you will notice them.

* Find music you love moving to, which you cannot stand still to, music with a strong beat that gets you going and play it when you exercise.

* Find a work-out partner, someone in the family, a girlfriend or a neighbour. Don't exercise alone if you can help it. You need someone so you can laugh, sweat and groan together. Make the session enjoyable. Create the fun factor. If you find a work-out buddy, always stick to your work-out time. Don't let them down.

* Finally, commit to exercising during a certain TV programme. I often exercise while watching the news before supper. You can only do this once you know my programme, but it works and time flies.

Some people suggest buying clothes a couple of sizes smaller. I actually think this is a demotivating ideal. It can seem unachievable when it can take quite sometime to get into a new dress size. Your choice of size may also be unrealistic.

I have a medical problem and do not think I can exercise.

Back pain is the most common. To be honest with you the right exercise can only help your health physically and mentally. Take time-out and talk in-depth to your doctor about your condition. Under medical advice and the guidance of a physiotherapist, take gradual steps to bring exercise into your life. For example, while back pain is often resolved by exercise, joint problems such as arthritis or osteoarthritis are more sensitive conditions, requiring trial and error to find out how long and hard you can exercise. If you have pain in the joints within two hours of exercise, you have worked-out too hard. Do not be put off. Exercise plays a vital role in health. Seek medical advice and build it in.

My body image is so low I feel too embarrassed to exercise in a class situation.

Feeling too embarrassed to go to exercise publicly because of your shape or size, because of how you see yourself is one of the biggest demotivators of all. You are not alone, most women I speak to and even

quite a few men have a low body image. This is something that cannot be resolved overnight but you can change your self-perception – exercise creates the feel-good factor almost instantly. The after-exercise high will boost your self-esteem, a higher self-esteem will lead to a commitment to one's self and lifestyle, and in turn you will change. When you exercise at home, no-one sees you, so do not be judgmental on yourself. Exercise in the baggiest of clothing, no-one is there to notice your shape or size.

It all seemed like too much hard work to get the results I want.

Results take time. There are no quick fixes when it comes to fat, weight loss or changing shape. The more exercise you do, the stronger you get, the more you can exercise, the more you do and the sooner you see results. The key to achieving your result is patience and perseverance.

I feel isolated working-out by myself. My family and partner laugh at me. They have always accepted me how I am, so why should I work-out?

This may be strange to say but sometimes people, work associates, your loved ones and friends do not want you to change. They can get jealous or afraid that you will be too attractive. They may tease you because they actually fear what the future may hold for you. How often have you heard girlfriends say when you have lost weight, 'You're getting too thin, don't lose any more'. It is strange. You were teased and made to feel bad when you were a cuddly, flabby person, but when it comes to change, often your partner and friends will not support you. This is when you need to take charge. Explain you want respect so that you do not feel you are on an uphill struggle to achieve the new you. Reassure them that this new you is not going to change your personality, you are still the same person inside. The new you will be a hell of a lot healthier and have more energy to cope with life. This new you may be sexier and more confident, and why not? The new you is far more likely to be fun-loving than depressed, down and lethargic. If your partner cannot cope with a new you and cannot support you as you change your lifestyle, then it is he or she who has a problem.

I stuck at the programme for ten weeks, saw results, felt good and then dropped the exercise habit. Now I have ended up regaining my original weight loss and more.

Basically, you cannot diet forever, you cannot exercise intensely and then think, 'I have lost weight, I have changed shape and now I can stop'. If you do not change your lifestyle and go back to your old habits, you will regain the weight.

The circumstances of my life changed. I moved (changed jobs, became ill, got pregnant, got married etc) and lost track of my programme. I have become a work-out stray with distant memories of being fit. I lost the self-discipline to stay on track. Being active was once no problem but now it is so easy to be distracted.

Get on target. I may not have all the answers but I intend to put you back on track using the positive powers of your mind to get you moving and sticking to your work-out. You have the power and total influence over yourself – not your friends, partner or coach – it is up to you to focus in and go for it. You have simply got to get back into the work-out habit.

* Focus on exercise memories – how it made you feel good after a work-out, how you felt in control, how things did not bother you so much and how stress was easier to handle.

* Do not focus on an old body shape when you may have been several kilos lighter and your body fat was lower.

* Set small goals. For ten minutes a day inch your way back to fitness.

* Being overenthusiastic will cause you to do too much too soon, risking injury.

* Gradually increase your workload by ten percent each week for five weeks, by then you should be back to your old routines.

* Your biggest effort will be to get up off the couch, away from the TV and to work-out.

* Do not let your mind talk you out of your work-out.

* Once you start don't compare your current fitness level with your old fitness levels.

* This is a sensitive time – keep positive. Mentally, state you are back in action. Be patient with yourself, it is going to take time to return to your old fitness levels.

* Focus on the moment when you are exercising. Focus on your breathing technique and how your muscles feel. At the end of the work-out focus on your achievement.

* Finally, be consistent in your training. Make the commitment to yourself so you re-establish the everyday work-out habit. Tell your family or partner what you are doing. Gradually increase training time as you gradually rebuild your strength, block out time in your work diary. Make an appointment with yourself. Remember: you come first, it is your body.

* If you have young kids who cannot amuse themselves, let them work-out next to you. If they get bored, have toys nearby. Allow them to create some mess, after the work-out you will have enough positive energy to both handle the mess and care for your kids.

* Make that appointment with yourself and stick to it.

I hate exercise, dieting is so much easier, but I never achieve permanent results.

This is a hard one, how can I tell you how to like exercise? It is impossible really to change your attitude but you know you should be doing something, otherwise you would not have got this far with the ULBT programme. Research has shown that the only way you will get permanent results is to combine regular exercise with a sensible, lifelong eating plan. Your mind has the power to change your attitude. The problem is that doing something you think you hate will always lead to failure because invariably you do not want to succeed. Learning something new is a challenge. The fear of not achieving your goals attributes to negative thoughts, especially if you have always been lazy. Since you left school, the thought of physical work and self-discipline seems horrifying. The only way to find enjoyment in exercise is to discover the feel-good factor.

One of the most motivating tips I can give you is that you do not need to train like an athlete. Exercise does not need to be exhausting to get results or to become enjoyable. Most people relate the word exercise with a super-fit, unobtainable, unrealistic image. You may have tried to get fit before by going to a class with your friends, but it was the wrong programme so it hurt. Everyone could do it but you. You hated the class, you felt embarrassed at your clumsiness, you hated feeling sore and in pain the next day. You hated the fact that your friends seemed to be fitter and had no problems when exercising. Turn this hate into self-discipline, change your attitude, go for it step-by-step. Getting fit and changing your shape does not need to hurt and it can be fun.

The following are some of the benefits of regular exercise. Knowing the benefits will help challenge your dislike, because how can you hate something that has proven health benefits, enhances your self-esteem, your looks and gives you the feel-good factor? If you hate the thought of the effort it takes, the latest research by Dr Rippe, Director of the Center for Clinical and Lifestyle Research, and Associate Professor of Medicine (Cardiology) at Tufts University School of Medicine (Boston, Massachusetts, USA) will encourage you.

At the end of 1995 he visited the UK to present an update on the world research on health and fitness. He talked about several studies relating to the health benefits of exercise.

I include extracts from his talk (with the courtesy of Forza Fitness Equipment who hosted his tour 'The Vision of The 90's) to help you understand why exercising regularly, being in shape and lowering your body fat is very important. Heart disease and cancer are one of the biggest concerns for most people and these were the main topics that were addressed.

Heart Disease

A major study was published in 1993 in the *New England Journal of Medicine* – "The Nurses Health Trial" – which followed over 100,000 nurses for over twenty years. If a woman gains over 10kgs or 22lbs beyond the age of eighteen, she increases her risk of heart disease by over 50 percent. Any time you gain a significant amount of weight it should raise the yellow caution flag. We, as a society, in both the UK and the USA are too fat. The fatter you are, the higher the risk of death from all causes.

In the USA a woman is six times more likely to die of heart disease than of breast cancer. When a woman becomes post-menopausal, she is ten times as likely to die of heart disease than of breast cancer. Heart disease is the number one cause of death in both men and women.

By being even a small amount overweight you increase the risk of heart disease and by the time you reach obesity, being 20 percent overweight, you increase your risk of heart disease by 50 percent. Even being just slightly over-weight significantly increases your risk of heart disease and cancer.

We have too many calories, our food chain has too much fat and alcohol in it and, most importantly, we lead increasingly sedentary lifestyles.

Unfortunately, the same problem is now occurring in children. It is increasing at about the same rate in children, which means that the problem we have in adults is small in comparison to the problem we will have in the next generation if we do not take very strong steps to make people understand that this a health problem and not a vanity problem. If obesity were an infectious disease, there would be national alarm bells sounding in the UK and USA, and yet, somehow, we have treated obesity as if it weren't a health problem at all. It is a health problem. It is of tremendous importance.

Cancer

In California, several thousand women who are moderate exercisers, exercising at a weekly level of about two to three hours of moderately intensive physical activity, were looked at over a number of years for any relationship between exercise and breast cancer. The results showed that women who exercise moderately for at least two hours a week reduce their risk of breast cancer by 50 percent.

What happens is that risk is mediated through body weight and exercise is associated with slightly lower body weight. Slightly lower body weight is associated with less oestrogen in the bloodstream and oestrogen plays a very important role in stimulating early phases of breast cancer. So, by exercising, women reduce the amount of circulating oestrogen in their bloodstream and thereby reduce the likelihood of developing breast cancer.

Nutrition & Cancer Prevention

The only practice where there is a universal agreement in terms of nutritional benefit, in terms of reducing your cancer risk, is to eat at least five servings of fruits and vegetables a day. It is the basis of the National Cancer Institute Programme 'Five Alive'.

The most important nutritional message we can get people to understand is that eating five servings of fruits and vegetables a day has been demonstrated to be the one nutritional practice that clearly lowers your risk of cancer. Probably because they have antioxidants, fibre and a bunch of other things that we still have not discovered.

Stress

Stress is an enormous problem in the USA. We estimate that approximately one-third of adults have enough stress in their work or private lives to hinder their performance. We need to find very easy, simple things that will help people deal with their stress.

We took highly anxious individuals and randomly assigned them either to a group which used a wireless heart rate monitor, or to a control group. These were highly anxious individuals. For the wireless heart rate monitor group the programme was very simple. We asked them to put on their heart rate monitor for ten minutes every day – only ten minutes – and to simply sit quietly and to try and pay attention to their heart rate with the idea of trying to slow it. Simply pay attention to your heart rate for ten minutes a day.

Those who did that had immediate, significant reductions in their anxiety and tension, and over a twelve-week period they actually changed the level of baseline anxiety in their life. They substantially improved their mood and quality of life. The group who did not use heart monitors were left to cope with stress in their own way. After a twelve-week period, the anxiety level in their life had not improved.

It is a very simple form of bio-feedback. We've tended to use bio-feedback in athletic performances but bio-feedback is terribly powerful in terms of stress reduction as well. Something so simple as paying attention to your heartbeat for ten minutes a day results in substantial stress reduction.

The basis of a stress-reduction programmes is to teach people to live in the here and now, not to fear the future or regret the past. Paying attention to your heart rate is one of the very powerful ways of getting a person to live in the here and now.

The future leads to creating exercise programmes that are age specific.

Dr James Rippe's words are extremely profound and vital for us to realize we need to take steps to be responsible for our present and future health.

THE BENEFITS OF EXERCISE

Do you really know the benefits of exercise? You may be surprised that there are at least fifty reasons why you should permanently make fitness part of your life.

Exercise & Your Body

Exercise:

- Strengthens the cartilage in joints
- Strengthens ligaments connecting bones and stabilizing joints
- Increases bone density
- Reduces the risk of developing osteoporosis
- Helps to slow down bone loss due to ageing
- Increases muscular strength and endurance
- Improves flexibility
- Makes the heartbeat stronger
- Improves the circulatory system
- Helps improve the condition of varicose veins
- Improves breathing and respiratory systems
- Can help alleviate asthma attacks
- Reduces the risk of heart disease
- Reduces the risk of developing cancer
- Assists with the discomfort of osteoarthritis
- Improves posture
- Helps strengthen the back and reduces lower-back pain
- Reduces PMS symptoms
- Reduces work absenteeism due to illness

Exercise & You

Exercise:

- Helps release stress
- Aids relaxation
- Reduces insomnia
- Increases daily energy levels
- Alleviates depression
- Improves self-esteem
- Reduces anxiety
- Improves body image
- Can help with eating disorders
- Can help to stop smoking
- Can stop alcohol and drug abuse of the body
- Improves the sex life
- Can help maintain a healthy diet
- Improves the complexion
- Slows down the ageing process
- Is one of the key factors for preventive health care
- Reduces visits to the doctor
- Reduces medical bills

Exercise & Weight

Exercise:

- Utilizes calories for energy
- Helps the body to burn energy
- Helps to reduce body-fat level and maintain lean body tissue
- Helps maintain body weight
- Helps temporarily reduce appetite
- Helps maintain a higher metabolic rate even when resting
- Improves the digestive system and alleviates constipation
- No creeping-weight syndrome due to ageing
- Helps improve cellulite

With these benefits in mind, what's stopping you? Especially when you thought that exercise was only for shaping up.

Make it work for you

Make it work for you

What does it take to get results? Three major steps. These are not simple changes, but once you have started, the process of change will escalate – your self-esteem will grow and grow and you will reach realistic goals.

Firstly, you need to assess your lifestyle, from your activity through to your eating habits. Throughout this book I have enclosed numerous assessment charts and work-out diaries to set you on the path to success. These are for your use only, a place where you can write down how you feel and be really honest with yourself. Even if you have not quite achieved your target one week, you will be able to see when you had really good or bad times and understand why.

The three vital steps to success are:

1. Develop a positive body image because your body image has a tremendous impact on permanent results. Once we accept ourselves we are able to take care of ourselves. Having a positive body image enables us to go for it and achieve realistic results.

2. Increasing activities is a vital factor. This doesn't mean you simply follow the ULBT programme three to five times a week, it means increasing your daily activity so that you are burning more calories. Walking daily, using the stairs, walking up the escalator, take up cycling, go dancing once a week, play squash, tennis and swim – it all adds up. Research has shown that those who live a more active lifestyle have the greatest chance for success.

3. Permanently change your regular eating habits. Following a strict, controlled diet leads to failure because you cannot diet for life – it is boring and tedious. Most dieters regain their weight loss once they've returned to their old eating habits. A permanent change doesn't mean you are on a diet for life, it means balance. The ULBT programme allows you to eat most things in moderation. There are no good foods or bad foods, no more guilt pangs, no more denial. Simply learn the art of nourishment, feeding your body and making balanced choices.

These three steps sound all too simple and, for some of you, too idealistic, since your lifestyle always turns stress into a negative state. During the next few chapters we are going to work at achieving your goals by self-monitoring. Your first step is to make a plan of change.

Your plan of change

Make a commitment to yourself and develop your lifetime achievement plan. Aim for simple changes in habit at first to prove to yourself you can make changes. You may want to fill this in now or after you've read the programme, but fill it in before you start the exercises.

My personal exercise goals will include regular aerobic activity as well as toning sessions:

1. _____

2. _____

3. _____

Examples

1. Brisk walk every day
2. Do ULBT on Monday, Wednesday, Friday and Sunday
3. Ride bike to work

In order to accomplish these I must do the following:

1. _____

2. _____

3. _____

Examples

1. Make time for myself
2. Walk in lunch hour
3. Find a work-out partner

My personal diet goals:

1. _____
2. _____
3. _____

Examples

1. Eat regularly
2. Eat less fat
3. Eat smaller portions

In order to accomplish these I must do the following:

1. _____
2. _____
3. _____

Examples

1. Eat breakfast
2. Stop buying chocolate
3. Eat with no distractions

My lifestyle goals:

1. _____
2. _____
3. _____

Examples

1. Leave work at 5.30pm
2. See a friend once a week
3. Relax more

In order to accomplish these I must do the following:

1. _____
2. _____
3. _____

Examples

1. Set alarm on watch
2. Phone old friends
3. Find out about stress release

My personal space goals:

1. _____
2. _____
3. _____

Examples

1. Have a weekly facial
2. I need more time to myself
3. Relax

In order to accomplish these I must do the following:

1. _____
2. _____
3. _____

Examples

1. Find a good beautician
2. Talk to partner/family about my needs
3. Get partner to massage me

Read this every week and tick your accomplishments. When you are down or disheartened with yourself, read it and remind yourself of what you have achieved. Rewrite your goals after six weeks or when you feel you can accomplish more. Do not forget this plan once you have achieved your goals. Every few weeks refer to it, even after a year look at it again and compare the new you to the old you. You will see a big difference!

How do you see yourself?

Maybe you are comfortable about yourself?
Maybe you cannot stop thinking about your body?

Examine your self-esteem by trying the body-image test.

Body-Image Test

1. Do you constantly worry about putting on weight or being fat?
   A Always
   B Sometimes
   C Never

2. When you think of your body shape do you focus on the parts you do not like ?
   A Always
   B Sometimes
   C Never

3. Is it hard for you to accept a compliment about how you are looking from your partner, family or friends?
   A Always
   B Sometimes
   C Never

4. Do you avoid doing activities where people will see your body, such as swimming, wearing fitted clothing in the park, an exercise class or at a party?
   A Always
   B Sometimes
   C Never

5. When was the last time you were happy about your weight?
   A Never
   B A few years ago before you had kids
   C Yesterday

6. Are you self-conscious about what you eat in front of people?
   A Always
   B Sometimes
   C Never

A: 5 Points
B: 3 Points
C: 1 Point
Add up your score.

20 – 30
You are rather hard on yourself. You need to make a conscious effort to develop yourself as number one. Read the body-image section often and take positive steps toward improving the way you see yourself. Remember you are unique and individual, so do not belittle yourself.

15 – 20
You are halfway to your goal. There are moments at which you appreciate yourself while at other times you are hard on yourself. Make an effort to be more positive and be aware of when you put yourself down.

Under 15
You have a positive body image. You do not let yourself get affected by things. You are one of the lucky ones. This is how we all want to be.

Body-Image

Looking back from my mid-teens and on into my twenties, the term 'body-image' did not exist. It was in the early Seventies that the USA medical profession began to connect eating disorders with body-image distortion. In my dancing days it was widely accepted that models and dancers simply did not eat. It was fashionable to live off coffee and cigarettes. Luckily I have never liked either so I ate and danced but what I ate was not predominately a healthy choice – most of us were chocaholics!

One of the main reasons we have a distorted body-image is because most of the images portrayed by the media are not realistic. Fashion models, who are genetically tall, long-limbed and, in most cases, beautiful, are 15 percent below their natural body weight. A vast number of actresses and TV presenters are underweight. The camera makes the body appear heavier on screen, so most celebrities are on never-ending diets to keep slim.

Back in the Seventies and the Eighties we had no idea that the influence of diet gurus, the fashion world, Jane Fonda and the media would have such an impact. Now we are all caught up in this world of poor self-esteem and distorted body-images from people aged sixty down to children of six.

So, why do we have this problem of poor body-image? Many people think that if they were taller or thinner or two stone lighter they would be happier, more successful or more loved. Most of us think if we could change in some way we would be a better person. The desire for physical perfection has spread in the West, causing us to look at imperfections, distorting our self-image and lowering our self-worth. The extreme problems of poor body-image lead to perpetual dieting and eating disorders, but it is possible to change and develop a healthier image by seeking expert medical help, professional counselling and by using methods of self-help.

You have the power within you to create a healthy body-image.

Learning to love and accept yourself and your imperfections will enable you to create a healthy body-image. This has a snowball effect, leading to success and long-term reality goals. By simply not being so hard on yourself or allowing in influences of the media and others, you will be able to take responsibility for your actions and lifestyle.

It all sounds so simple but it isn't. How you see and treat yourself is unique. There are so many ingrained reasons why you have low self-esteem and a poor body-image.

What I am going to do is to try and put the way you see yourself into perspective and then it is up to you to decide that you are going to take responsibility for yourself. This may mean seeking expert help, or it may mean facing up to situations or an issue with someone that you may have been trying to avoid.

Firstly, I want you to realize that you are not alone and if you took time to ask your friends and work colleagues how they see themselves, you'd find that most have a poor body-image of themselves as well. So, let's get this body-image problem into proportion.

Body-image – words stick, let's change them.

What do you imagine when you think of the word 'thin'? I instantly have a picture of Kate Moss in my mind. Most of us relate the word to supermodels who are not a realistic image.

What do you think of when you see or hear the word 'weight'? Do you instantly focus on yourself or think of dieting? What celebrity do you visualize?

From my own research, I have found that most of us relate any conversation that includes the word 'weight' to ourselves. Mentally, we focus on our worst bits, the size of our thighs, tums or whatever. We automatically enhance and create our own negative body image.

The next time you start being hard on yourself, criticizing your shape and pulling your body to bits, stop and change this negative thinking into positive. It may sound crazy but trying saying to yourself 'I do not look like Marlon Brando or 'Carry On' star Hattie Jacques, I am me and I am doing OK, in time I'm going to be healthier, fitter and firmer'. This may sound silly but you are creating an affirmation and by saying it aloud to yourself each day, whenever you are triggered into thinking about weight, actually helps towards turning negative thinking into positive thinking. It is a fun way of putting your own body-image into perspective.

Avoid berating yourself every time you look in a mirror.

Your brain is a living computer, so stop feeding it negative information about your shape, be aware of what you call yourself. Stop saying 'fat' and replace it with a word such as 'curvy'.

Do not allow the scales to rule your life.

Throw them away, especially if you are weight fixated. Every time you get on those scales you are putting your self-esteem to the test. More often than not you are disappointed, wishing you had not indulged in 'that chocolate bar' the night before. Most weight charts are inaccurate anyway. Targeting yourself on a set weight is a mistake.

Remember:

▷ If you are a woman, your weight will vary throughout your monthly cycle due to hormonal changes.

▷ Your weight is not the issue, it is your body density that matters – the amount of lean body tissue you have compared to your body fat.

▷ Some of you will even gain muscle weight yet lose inches as you become leaner, while the fat cells shrink and your muscle mass increases

through the regular work-outs

▷ Measure your progress by how you feel, how your clothes fit and how you look.

I've included a progress monitoring chart to use on page 26. This is a great way to monitor the changes in your body but remember, even using a tape measure the measurement will vary unless you always measure yourself under the same circumstances. This means the same time of day and the same day of the week. Women need to allow for variation due to monthly cycles.

▷ In the USA, a national organization for eating disorders, awareness and prevention uses the slogan, 'Do not Weigh Your Self-esteem'.

▷ Stop singling out the bits you do not like about yourself, accept that you are a whole person, you can't go through life hating parts of your body. Emphasize your most attractive parts, whether it's your bust, legs or knees, and accept the rest.

▷ Do not get disturbed by media images of the supermodels. Learn to look at them in a different way. Look artisically at the styling, the photography and the make-up, not at the size of the model.

▷ If you are feeling down about your shape, go to the local leisure centre and look at all the differently shaped bodies in the pool. These are reality images.

Never forget:

The models and actresses you see do not look the way they do without expert help and perfect lighting. They can afford personal trainers and long gym sessions. The rest of us have the real world to cope with – jobs, responsibilities, studying and making ends meet – so do not be hard on yourself. Allow yourself to accept and enjoy yourself.

I recently yelled out on the microphone when I was teaching a LBT session at Fit'n'Fun to over a thousand people, 'We are not the Claudia Schiffers of this world, we are reality and you look great!' The crowd laughed and when later during the session I asked them, 'What are you?' they yelled back, 'Reality and great'. The laughter and energy was electric. These people, women and men of all ages, were accepting themselves, they had the same aim to get the most out of their lives.

At the end of the session a young woman approached me and in a very quiet voice said, 'I have been coming to you for three years now. I have followed your exercise video and because of you I was inspired to lose eleven stone.' She was nearly in tears and so was I. She is an amazing individual who has reached her goal (you can read her story at the end of the book).

Research has shown that in the younger generation, children as young as five are diet-conscious. Body-image and eating-disorder problems are often passed down from parent to child. Be aware of this if you are a parent. Do not make critical comments about your child's physical appearance, their body or how they look. Do not let your child hear you criticize yourself or your friends' shapes. Talk to your partner, make them aware that teasing or openly showing disappointment about shape, size or features will establish a pattern of poor self-esteem, body-image and a future of dieting. It could even lead to eating disorders.

Do not bring attention to your child's diet. The easiest and simplest way to create healthy eating patterns is not to have food battles but to cook together, to make food choices together and not make a big issue out of fattening foods.

Having four daughters has been a real education for me regarding how they see themselves, each other and how they make food choices. They were all brought up on ultra-healthy diets when they were babies but that does not control their food choices or eating habits as they grow. Today, they all have a healthy attitude to themselves and their food. We

have had our moments but we have always talked over the issue.

Fitness instructors obviously have to teach a lot and look good, but often the physical image of an instructor distorts your goals. Their lifestyle is totally different from yours. The majority of fitness instructors exercise two to three times a day. Many also do their own training of some kind. It is a well-known, worldwide fact in the industry that a vast majority of fitness instructors have an eating disorder of some sort, because even those who expose their shape to the public eye day-in and day-out have a poor body-image. The hard-bodied, ultra-toned muscular look is what most instructors strive for, and some will do anything to achieve it.

In some countries instructors have to have this look to get a teaching job. To have an ultra-lean body look, one's body fat has to be very low, usually below 17 percent. This is unrealistic and unhealthy as the National Exercise for Life Institute's recommendation for a woman's body fat is between 20–25 percent. In some cases it can be detrimental to the health to have such a low body fat. Infertility and osteoporosis are the biggest problems within the teaching industry. Many teachers have spent years overtraining and dieting. Basically, you've been conned. The image of an instructor you see in class is not reality. Going to a class or following a programme because you're inspired by the instructor's physique is an impossible goal unless you work-out for three hours a day.

When you work through the exercise sequences, you will see a variety of body shapes in the models, including myself and two of my daughters. Everyone is a different shape. Whether you are short and stocky like myself or tall and long-limbed like my model Katie J, you too can look good. You may have seen her in my videos, she's always there! This is because we are total opposites in build.

I've illustrated the exercises with a variety of body shapes because I've seen so many fitness books where beautiful professional ultra-lean models of 5ft 10in have been used, creating a false image. Most of these photographic models have never worked-out and they lack the muscle tone and shape of a fit body. My programme is about reality – the models are real and they all have healthy, fit bodies.

Here is a picture of me when I taught five hours a day and was running two of London's major fitness clubs. In those days I was a single parent with three kids and yes, I was lean but I had no bust and a low sex drive. I was always suffering from an injury. I taught twenty-five classes a week for four-and-a-half years until one day I collapsed from exhaustion and was put to bed for a total rest – my body had burnt out.

I am curvier now and several years older. I have had to come to terms with the fact that I cannot train or teach like I used to. I have had to face the fact that after the birth of my fourth daughter late in life I have ended up with a weight problem. Apparently, every time you are pregnant you lay down more fat cells, it is nature's way of creating fat storage for breast-feeding. I have been pregnant six times, so my metabolic rate and fat cells have had a hey-day!

These days I am very busy but for most of my time I am sitting in meetings or at my desk all day. I have not accepted this quietly and I have been inwardly so angry that I am no longer totally in control of my body. I cannot take three hours out of a day to train. Many a time when I am about to go off to train, a major drama will erupt at home and I choose to stay. I am a working mum whose quality time with her family is precious. Kids grow up so fast and then they go, leaving home to get on with their own lives. I have to be around for my responsibilities! My situation is not unique, it is reality. My message is all about reality – to find your realistic shape and achieve your realistic goals, to be the ultimate you. This is not an overnight process.

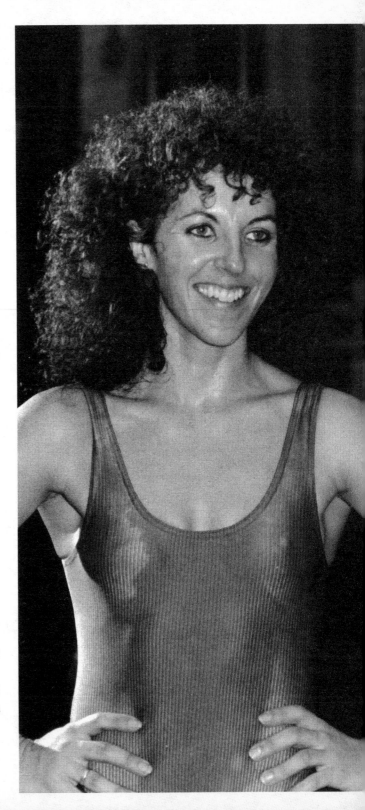

The Ultimate Legs Tums 'N' Bums Personal Monitoring Chart

Monitor your weekly progress. Don't be disheartened if you don't see an immediate transformation.
It takes time to achieve a permanent shape change.
Remember this is a plan for a healthier and fitter lifestyle, so be strong and stick with it!

Questions	Example	Week 1	Week 2	Week 3	Week 4	Week 5	Week 6	Week 7	Week 8	Week 9	Week 10
How often did you exercise this week?											
Aerobic beginner	4										
Aerobic Advanced	6										
ULBT beginner	3										
ULBT Advanced	5										
How did you feel after exercising?											
Great	Y										
Exhausted											
Relaxed	Y										
Re-energized	Y										
How do you feel this week?											
Moody											
Tired											
Bored											
Just coping											
Relaxed											
Good	Y										
Energized											
Fine											
In control											
Ready for anything											

Continued on next page

Questions	Example	Week 1	Week 2	Week 3	Week 4	Week 5	Week 6	Week 7	Week 8	Week 9	Week 10
What are your measurements?											
Bust	38										
Waist	36										
Hips	38										
Left arm	17										
Right arm	18										
Left thigh	22										
Right thigh	23										
Eating – how was the week for you?											
Fine											
Controlled											
Planned											
Less fatty foods	Y										
More fruit											
More fish	Y										
More fresh veg											
Hopeless											
Binged											
Stressed											
Couldn't be bothered											
PMS eating											
Take-aways											
Too sociable											
Too much sweet food											
Too much dairy produce											

Always try to measure yourself with the same tape measure, if this is not possible,
use tight-fitting clothing to see if there are any differences.

Diets are out

YOU HAVE TRIED THEM ALL BUT WONDER WHY YOU STILL DO NOT LOOK HOW YOU WANT TO... DIETS ARE OUT.

Almost everyone, whatever their background, social status and income, is aware of dieting and thinks about or tries to lose weight sometime in their life. To be blunt, we are diet obsessed. Everyone wants instant weight loss but fat cannot dissolve overnight or melt away through using pills, creams or body wraps. Even so, this does not stop most dieters from trying every fad diet possible in the hope of instant results.

For some, losing weight has become their sole aim in life. For many others it is a ritual eating plan that they implement after festive times such as Christmas. There are dietholics who buy every possible diet book and gimmick around in the hope that it is going to be the answer to shifting their excess weight. Dieting is a multi-million pound business that affects us all.

You may think you are in control when you diet but read the following points and consider. Are you really in control or is the diet in control of you?

Diet Points

▶ Healthy eating has been promoted for over twenty years but we are still a fat nation.

▶ Anyone can suffer from an eating disorder, not just celebrities.

▶ You are in a high-flying job. Everyone around you is ultra-thin and fashion conscious. You simply have to diet.

▶ You are dieting so you put your whole family on a diet.

▶ Every day you look in the mirror and say, 'If I lose a few pounds, I'll be happier, successful, beautiful...'

▶ You lose weight but you are still unhappy. Inside you feel fat.

▶ You look at others eating and think, 'How can they eat whatever they like?' – when you simply cannot.

▶ You decide to diet before you attempt to put on work-out gear and go to class.

▶ Do you intend to diet for life? If so why? You are caught in a vicious diet trap, always feeling hungry and disliking yourself.

▶ You are too thin. You think you are in control of your body but your body is in control of you.

▶ You lose weight for a while – then you regain it – and more.

▶ You cannot stop thinking about fattening foods.

▶ You do not go out and socialize because you are on a diet.

▶ You are so preoccupied with food and dieting that there is no time for anything else.

▶ You are always on a diet.

▶ A good diet means healthy, nutritional eating – not starving yourself.

▶ You are overweight and in emotional pain and find it hard to break the cycle of bingeing, yo-yo dieting and bulimia.

▶ Our lifestyles, our daily stress and our upbringing have turned us into diet freaks.

▶ You turn the lights off when you undress in front

of your partner because you feel fat and ashamed of your body.

▶ A balanced diet means eating from all the food groups.

▶ What happened to the family meal?

▶ What happened to home cooking?

▶ We all know what we should eat but we do not do it.

▶ What happened to a balanced diet?

▶ What happened to simply enjoying food?

▶ What happened to feasting for celebration where you could eat without feeling guilty?

▶ You have dieted so much you lost weight as well as your sex drive, periods and breast tone.

▶ You simply do not have time to eat properly.

▶ Fast foods, high in fat, high in sugar are comfort foods. Stress-related foods are our main source of nourishment.

FROM DIETING TO EATING DISORDERS

Extreme dieting leads to eating disorders. The ultimate eating disorder is anorexia, when the person attempts to control their weight by simply starving themselves.

Anorexia and bulimia are words that fly around flippantly these days but it is important that we all face the fact that diet-mania has been created through the belief that being thin is beautiful. Lack of self-esteem has caused such poor body-image. Many people have eating disorders of some kind.

Anorexia Nervosa

This is defined as a psychological eating disorder. An anorexic is a person who intentionally starves themselves.

People often assume that anorexia is related to women who are obsessed with losing weight and are narcissistic about their bodies. Anorexics are usually in emotional torment. Many have a history of emotional or sexual abuse which has never been resolved; experiences that may have started as a young child or in puberty. Some cases are related to high-pressure stress levels or the result of a painful relationship.

What is common for all anorexics is that they feel inhuman. Their self-esteem is nil and their body image is totally distorted. People can die from anorexia, or be scarred for life by osteoporosis or infertility. I have never been anorexic but I've had close friends who have suffered from it. It is one of the saddest, self-inflicted diseases there is. If you know someone close to you who is anorexic or if you are yourself, please seek help (see Useful Addresses).

Bulimia

A bulimic has an irresistible urge to eat without restraint, triggered by particular moods, events, stress or circumstance. Drastic efforts are used to counteract the effect of the binge from self-induced vomiting, laxatives, diuretics and other drugs to complete starvation. Bingeing is not uncommon. Everyone I know binges at sometime, whether it is a food or drink binge, overeating at a meal or in private, or PMS bingeing on food because you love the taste. The enjoyment of a food binge is totally different from out-of-control stress bingeing (where you do not taste what you eat). Bulimia is the expunging of the food you have secretly stuffed yourself with in order to avoid weight gain, or to eliminate the fullness by vomiting and using an excessive amount of laxatives. Bulimia is a complicated eating disorder, and there is more than one type of bulimia.

Bulimia Nervosa

This has always been reported as an eating disorder related to anorexia. Bulimia Nervosa occurs when the key symptoms of anorexia – severe persistent loss of weight and the absence of monthly periods – have subsided. What continues is the fear of calories and fat – enter Bulimia Nervosa.

Bulimarexia

This can be part of Anorexia Nervosa. An estimated 50 percent of established anorexics binge from time to time. What they eat may not be excessive but they still vomit as part of the constant effort of dieting to remain in control.

Normal Weight Bulimia (NWB)

This is when bulimia occurs without being anorexic. The person's body weight is near normal or above.

Binge-Eating Disorder

This is the unrestrained eating that is so similar to bulimia but the person does not panic with guilt afterwards. This person does not vomit to get rid of the food as long as there is no huge increase in weight. It becomes habitual if there are emotional or relationship problems affecting work or social life. Binge-eating is now considered to be part of the same disorder as bulimia. A binge-eater can become a bulimic when they discover an immediate release from vomiting.

Abnormal Weight Control Syndrome

This is predominantly a female problem. The girl or woman feels fat even if she is of normal weight. She panics and starves, vomits or purges herself, even if she has not overeaten. She is then ravenously hungry and starts to binge – enter the vicious circle of bulimia.

FACT:

90 percent of bulimics are women in their twenties. 10 percent are male in the same age group. Bulimia is rare in Afro-Caribbean or Asian communities.

Eating disorders are not something you simply brush aside or accept. Whether you, or someone close to you, binges, vomits or starves, the reality is that help is needed. Eating disorders comprise anorexia, bulimia and obesity. Most obese people hide away from the public eye, existing in a very inactive and lonely world.

FACT:

Over five million adults in the UK are obese. Recent Government statistics show that the prevalence of clinical obesity is doubling each decade.
The USA rate of obesity is much higher than in the UK and is rising.

The Health of the Nation Targets

By the year 2005, to reduce the proportion of obese people from:
MEN: 13 percent to 6 percent
WOMEN: 16 percent to 8 percent

Treatment that could be a way forward in terms of obesity therapy include:

1 Keeping a continual diary of bingeing and eating habits for clinical reference.
2 Identifying the weight cycle and then understanding and accepting that short-term weight loss cannot be sustained.
3 For long-term benefits, weight maintenance may be more important than the effects of yo-yo dieting and weight fluctuation.
4 Reducing health risk should also be a priority, weight loss should not be the only goal.
5 Designing physical activity to motivate and give results for obese clients.
6 An understanding of the appearance-related problems suffered by the obese, from body image to society's reaction towards them.
7 Understanding that obesity is not a simple

problem of overeating.

8 The importance of social support.

9 Understanding that change can only happen when the patient is ready to adopt positive lifestyle and behaviour patterns.

10 Recognizing that although there are many self-help manuals and a wide range of professionals catering for the obese, no two people are alike and what works for one may not work for another.

11 The importance of health education in schools and throughout the media in preventing future obesity.

It is time the fitness world created programmes that really do cater for the obese. As a fitness professional, my vision for 2005 would be the development of centres which combine nutrition and exercise programmes for everyone, and are run jointly with doctors, nutritionists and down-to-earth, un-intimidating qualified fitness instructors. Dieting is the weight war. The only way to win is breaking the habit through education and support groups. This means sorting out the reasons why you need to diet, starve yourself or binge.

Many fit cynics state that you have a problem because you simply eat too much and are not active enough. Their answer is simple! But is it really? There are so many social, lifestyle, emotional and genetic reasons for our national weight problem, yet the main reason is dieting and inactivity.

So, what does one do? Rebel and throw all dieting to the wind? Decide that life is worth living, you will stay fat, eat what you like and try to love yourself? It is not quite that simple. Very few of us can accept ourselves this way. There are also major health considerations – do you really want to invite a heart attack?

The key is to take responsibility for yourself. Taking responsibility means taking the steps to seek help – whether it is via a therapist, support group or your family – do something.

The Weight War

During my research for this book and as editor of *Get Active* magazine, I have had the opportunity to interview world experts on weight loss and health issues. What fascinates me now is that all the recent research has proven that the combination of regular exercise and good nutrition is the lifelong key to successful weight management. The following are extracts from my recent interview with an expert I greatly admire, Dr Daniel Kosich, who is the consulting senior director for the professional development at IDEA, president of EXERFIT Lifestyle Consulting in Denver, Colorado and is technical advisor to Jane Fonda Health and Fitness. He has spent fifteen years working with clients who wanted to, or needed to, lose some weight. I found his answers fascinating, which is why I want to share them with you.

Why do diets not work as a permanent answer to weight loss?

Mostly because the body needs an adequate amount of the nutrients, or energy, we get from food to work most efficiently. When we do not eat enough on a regular basis, our body tries to adjust. Sooner or later the body's demand for food prevails and the diet is abandoned. It is kind of like trying to hold your breath. You can hold it for a while, but before long you simply have to breathe again.

For a long time in the fitness world, instructors have advocated low-impact, long-duration aerobic exercise for the most effective fat-burning form of exercise. Now there is a swing back to high-impact, high-intensity, shorter duration aerobic exercise.
What is your opinion?

The key to burning the most fat is to burn the most calories. Those in poor condition need to work at a low intensity for a longer duration in order to burn a lot of calories. If they try to work at a high intensity, they will fatigue quickly, limiting total calorie burning. But as one's fitness level improves, it is possible to work harder, burning a lot more calories every minute, without rapidly fatiguing, so the duration can be shortened without limiting calorie burning. Those in poor condition do not have this option. The bottom line is that if I want to lose a pound of fat this week, I need to burn about 3,500 more calories than I take into my body. It does not really matter how I burn those calories. The harder, the longer and the more often I can exercise, the greater is the calorie burning.

Do you think certain body types or shapes have a tendency to put on weight or do they genetically have more fat cells?

I think the research clearly suggest that there is some genetic component to the whole spectrum of issues which impact weight management. Some people do have more fat cells than others. And there are also lots of different body shapes. It is not body shape which influences gaining weight. However, gaining or losing body weight is related to energy balance – calories in versus calories out. Those who have a naturally higher metabolic rate can eat more calories without gaining weight.

Do fat cells increase in women as they age?

Theoretically, in both men and women, the number of fat cells on the body is set by the time we reach adulthood. However, in both men and women (fat cells are the same in either gender), new fat cells can be made even as adults if they become big enough. If excess fat is stored, first, the cells that exist become bigger and bigger. Then, at some critical size (threshold size), the fat cell divides into two smaller cells, increasing the total number of fat cells.

There is a trend for women to have babies later in life. Many of these women now have a weight problem due to late motherhood. What is your opinion?

Weight problems following pregnancy are not limited just to those women who have babies later in life. The reasons are not totally clear. Some researchers attribute it to physiological changes associated with the so-called 'weight control set-point'. If a woman gains a lot of weight during pregnancy, there is also the possibility that new fat cells could be made. Lifestyle changes following pregnancy, such as less activity and/or more dietary calories, are also an issue in many cases. In my opinion, there are undoubtedly a myriad of factors which are involved, at any age. Regardless of what occurs in a woman that makes weight control more difficult following pregnancy, weight management is still an issue of calorie balance. Try to get more active to burn more calories, and eat a sensible diet.

How can you have two sisters with the same parents and genes, one of whom has never had a weight problem, the other one who has, when they live in the same household, both are active in sports and fitness and they eat the same foods in identical quantities?

Siblings do not have the same genetic make-up, unless perhaps they are identical twins. An offspring's genetics are a result of the multitude of possible combinations of the mother's and father's genetic make-up. While siblings may share a few or several genetic characteristics, we are all uniquely individual.

There is a strong emphasis from nutritionists to lower one's daily fat intake to a certain level, with an emphasis on increasing one's

carbohydrate intake for energy.

Can you put on weight by eating too many carbohydrates?

Weight gain occurs when calorie intake is greater than calorie expenditure, regardless of the source of calories – whether it be fats, carbohydrates or protein. The American Dietetics Association recommends that not more than 30 percent of daily calories come from fat. (The gram intake would be 30 percent of whatever the daily calorie intake is). About 55–60 percent of calories should come from carbohydrates, the remainder from protein. The suggestion that such a carbohydrate intake will lead to hyperinsulinemia, and therefore, an increase in body fat is not supported by the vast majority of international research. Hyperinsulinemia is more likely the result of carrying too much body fat, which in the USA is about 33 percent of the adult population.

Are there foods that speed up or stimulate one's metabolic rate?

It depends on what you mean. Yes, calories are burned when fats, carbohydrates and proteins are digested and absorbed. It 'costs' more to digest a protein and carbohydrate than it does fat. This is called the 'thermic effect of digestion', and accounts for about 10 percent of a person's daily calorie expenditure. Research has not discovered any foods which will help increase the burning of fat. Nicotine, caffeine, ephedrine and many other agents are stimulants, but their impact on increasing metabolic rate with regard to weight control is of little consequence. Eating this pill or this food and burning more calories while you sleep is an exciting fantasy.

Should women reassess their eating habits as they age?

One of the key dietary concerns with ageing, in both genders, is eating enough food and drinking enough water. Older people are more prone to dehydration. Many people experience a decrease in appetite as they get older. Inadequate calorie intake not only impacts energy levels, but also leads to nutrient deficiencies. For example, it is difficult to get enough calcium when the daily calorie intake is less than 1,200 calories. The guidelines for sensible eating apply at any age. However, following menopause, a woman should increase her calcium intake if she chooses not to go on oestrogen replacement.

Many people talk about slow metabolism as being a cause for their weight problem. Does a slower metabolism increase one's weight problem?

A naturally slower metabolism (resting metabolic rate) is part of the energy expenditure side of the equation. It does not automatically increase the potential for weight problems. The balance between calories in and calories out applies regardless of resting metabolic rate. Those with slower resting rates often simply need to get more active – burn more calories – to effectively balance the energy equation.

Why do people plateau when losing weight?

Nobody knows for sure. But it is likely to be related to metabolic adjustments the body makes. A lot depends on how the weight is lost. Low-calorie diets often result in a weight-loss plateau in a week or two, most likely the result of an acute decrease in resting metabolic rate (part of the set-point theory). Plateaux are much less likely when the weight loss occurs as a result of increasing calorie expenditure through exercise.

OUT-OF-CONTROL EATING

Before you make changes to your choice of food, let's look at your eating habits.

Do you suffer from out-of-control eating habits, overeating because you have a stressful life, are bored or simply love food? I am not talking about eating disorders, the following out-of-control eating patterns can occur from lifestyle habits which you can change when you understand why.

Problem

You simply cannot stop eating once you start. You usually miss breakfast and start to eat from midday until bedtime.

Why

You are not eating often enough. Starving yourself until midday, when your blood-sugar level has really dropped from the binge last night, creates excessive hangover.

Solution

Eat three meals and two snacks a day. Feed your body so that you do not eat excessively once you start to eat.

Problem

You cannot stand breakfast, manage to eat a sandwich at lunch time, but feel sleepy around 4pm so you grab something sweet. Re-energized, you want more sweet foods. You feel relaxed in the evening but you eat non-stop.

Why

It is the same problem. The body is desperate for food but because you ate high-calorie fatty foods late at night, you cannot face breakfast and start the day with just coffee. Grabbing a chocolate bar at 4pm gives you a quick lift then a rapid energy let down. When you are at home you consume a vast amount of food to make up for the calorie loss during the day.

Solution

Re-educate your taste buds and brain. Have fruit for breakfast even if it is just a banana before you rush off to work or do the school run. Eat less and plan your meal at night. Fill up on protein and vegetables and avoid high-fat starchy biscuits or chocolates. Do not eat after 8pm. Within a week you will be happily eating breakfast because you will be waking up hungry. Eat healthy snacks such as fruit and nuts.

Problem

Eating out all the time or with friends and family. You always overindulge.

Why

This is difficult because you do not want to be antisocial, but research has shown that the more people at the table the more food you eat. You will eat faster depending on the atmosphere, often not even being aware of the amount eaten.

Solution

If you find it impossible to eat well and with control when you are with your family and friends, eat alone for a while. Do not allow food to be the main social part of your life. Warn your family or partner that you need to get in control of your eating. Food is not going to be so important for you. Plan other activities where you can all do something together.

Problem

It is tough standing in front of a stove cooking. You simply cannot cook without tasting.

Why

All your senses are stimulated as you cook. It is difficult to cook without tasting if you are hungry.

Solution

Have something to eat before you cook – try fruit or drink a tomato juice. Then try and have help while you cook so you talk more and taste less. Do not clear away. Ask someone else to do this part. All the leftovers should be binned or frozen. Cook less so there aren't any leftovers.

Problem

You can eat really sensibly in front of people but on your own you binge. No-one sees you, so you stuff yourself with your favourite foods. You eat fast and furiously, not really tasting the food because you are worried you may be caught.

Why

This may be due to behavioural patterns. Were you educated about food as a child or are you pressurized by friends and family to be thin? Social eating does not encourage overindulging. You often see men tucking into a hearty meal but the pressure is on women to eat little and never overindulge. You do not want anyone to comment on your eating so you turn to eating in secret.

Solution

Check out why you are stressed. Something is bothering you. The food is a comfort for you. It may be a habit ingrained when you were a child longing for affection, or you may have always been rewarded by food. Think back, think why this happens but do not be angry with yourself.

Problem

You simply love food and have always been able to eat everything without having a weight problem, up until now.

Why

Most people have a variable, healthy appetite which can vary depending on anything from climate changes to energy expenditure. The body is an amazing machine that copes with most things in life but there comes a point when it says enough is enough. Usually over thirty and especially around mid-life.

Solution

You need to reassess your eating habits and diet.

Reduce your fat, sugar and alcohol intake. Still enjoy food but learn to moderate. Become more active, take up regular, aerobic, calorie-burning exercise so that your metabolic rate and digestion improves. As you age you may need to aid your digestion with a digestive enzyme supplement; seek advice from a nutritionist.

Problem

You are a plus size and feel you will never change. Your whole family have always been overweight, you love to binge, why change?

Why

You think that because you were born heavy, you will always be heavy, but this will only be true if throughout your life you have always been overfed and inactive. Genes have a lot to do with heavier builds. I've had four children, all heavy babies at birth, and the heaviest at birth is now the thinnest. Food is not important to her. She won't have a weight problem unless what she eats does not balance with her energy output.

Solution

You can decide to stay this way but you are leading up to a future full of health problems. Over 60 percent of the population in this country are overweight. Make the decision to change your diet to lose weight for a future of happy health. Do it slowly and patiently, take regular exercise. Even half an hour of daily brisk walking and a sensible healthy diet will transform your lifestyle completely.

Problem

Your diet is fine until ten days before your period. Then you lose complete control and binge on sweet, stodgy, fried food. Once your period starts, everything settles down and you are in control again. Every month you say to yourself next time it will not happen, that you will stay in control, but every month it always does!

Why

Premenstrual overeating is seen as a normal part of a woman's cycle and is accepted as being part of PMS. But it is a woman's nightmare because the body craves for junk food and it is very easy to binge at this time. The body actually needs more calories around the time of your period, which is why one has bouts of uncontrolled eating. It seems to get worse with age and stress. It is all blamed on hormones. The rapid rise of the female sex hormone oestrogen affects neurotransmitters and there is often a slight increase in weight at this time. The premenstrual weight gain is lost almost immediately after the period. Taking supplements can help control bingeing but seek professional help from your doctor or nutritionist. During this period do not condemn yourself for bingeing. Allow it, enjoy it and be free of guilt.

Solution

Eat small, frequent, starchy meals to reduce sugar cravings. This may mean every three hours and six snacks a day. Choose foods such as whole grains, bananas, nuts, seeds, vegetables (cooked or raw) and fruit. Avoid salty junk foods, sweets, cakes, pastries, sugary cereal, biscuits, chocolate and white bread. This will help to reduce water retention. Reduce your alcohol intake dramatically as alcohol often interferes with blood-sugar levels. Ensure that your food intake is little and often. This also helps keep blood-sugar levels even.

Eat foods that are high in potassium, a mineral that helps alleviate water retention, such as vegetables, bananas, carrots, cauliflower (preferably raw), leeks, endive, lentils (which are especially high in potassium), chicken and lean meat.

The urge to binge can be too tough so opt for low-fat foods such as popcorn, really fresh bread or exotic fruits. Have your diet checked with a nutritionist, you may need to take a multivitamin and mineral supplement plus Evening Primrose oil (a form of GLA essential fatty acid). Be patient, it takes as long as two to three months for supplements to have an effect on the body.

Problem

You drive a lot because of work or lifestyle demands but you cannot drive for long without wanting to eat something. Often after a long drive you cannot stop eating. You hate long journeys because you eat so much junk.

Why

Driving takes intense concentration. Even if you feel relaxed and in control it is a stressful situation. Eating sweet food or chocolate stimulates the blood sugar, and in theory your concentration, due to the rapid rise in blood sugar. Unless you are being distracted by talking to somebody, which is not always advisable when driving, you simply want something to chew on. This leads to sweet stuffing.

Solution

Do not drive on an empty stomach, have food before your journey, take healthier snack options, plus coffee and water. Chewing gum is a low-calorie solution. Avoid those huge bags of sweets and chocolate at the service station.

Problem

New mothers who managed throughout their pregnancy to maintain a healthy weight often find they put on weight when breast-feeding because they cannot stop eating when feeding.

Why

Firstly, nursing mothers are using up more calories, so in a perfect world, if the mother kept to a perfect diet, she would actually lose weight and regain her figure. Motherhood is stressful. One's hormones and blood-sugar levels fluctuate rapidly during this time. At feeding time women often feed themselves on biscuits or sugary snacks while feeding baby, or during those long wakeful nights, will eat out of boredom or desperation. Thirst is often replaced by food not fluid.

Solution

Adjusting to motherhood is not easy. Outwit yourself
with food. Only have healthy food options in the
house such as fruit for late-night snacks. Drink
plenty of mineral water before eating, at least one
and a half litres a day. During those quiet feed times
read a good book, avoid aimlessly watching TV and
putting food into your mouth. Breast-feeding burns
up calories so if you can control your food choices
and maintain a healthy calorie intake, those excess
fat stores will be utilized, especially when combined
with regular exercise, leaving you a slimmer self
once you have stopped feeding.

STRESS EATING

Anyone can react to a stress and overeat, not
occasionally, but several times a week. Whatever
the reasons for stress, good or bad, one often eats
to reward and comfort one's self, especially with
junk foods. Comfort eating is one of the main
causes of weight gain and it is something that most
of us suffer from.

How to handle stress eating

Stress depletes certain vitamins and minerals. At
stressful times make an effort to eat real foods. Plan
a meal that contains vegetables and proteins such
as meat or eggs. If you do not have time to eat,
avoid grabbing the nearest chocolate or cake. Drink
a low-fat, low-sugar milkshake or eat a handful of
almonds or a mix of sunflower, pumpkin and
sesame seeds. These foods are high in the nutrients
which are depleted when one is under stress.

Classic stress-eating situations

1   You have just arrived home and all you want to
    do is eat. It is as though your home environment
    is the trigger for you to eat, because you are in
    your comfort zone. Make sure you eat properly
    during the day. Snack on fruit when you are
    travelling home so you do not raid the fridge the
    moment you get in.

2   You are tired and you think that eating will re-
    energize you. Why not re-energize with exercise,
    spend time with a friend or read a good book?

3   You are too tired to cook so you order a take-
    away. Keep delicious, low-fat, ready-made,
    healthier meals in the fridge. Avoid that take-
    away.

4   You had a tough day, nothing worked out so you
    eat to de-stress. When this happens, exercise
    first to get rid of the negative stress. Then eat
    and you will be in control.

Eat a proper meal as soon as you can without distractions, and plan what you will eat. At least once a week find another form of stress release such as massage, having a facial or taking up yoga or meditation – sleep is one of the best stress releases. Take ten minutes out of your day to sit quietly and focus on yourself, your breathing and your heartbeat.

If your stress eating is turning into something far deeper, far too powerful for you to handle, seek help. I'm not a psychologist, this is not my area. I can only support you by telling you to speak to an expert in this field. Do not, however, abandon exercising as it is one of the few sources of positive activity you can do.

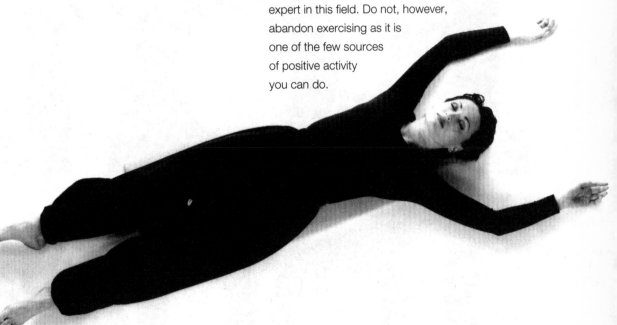

Eat to Tone

EAT FOR ENERGY ▶ EAT FOR HEALTH ▶ EAT FOR LIFE

We all want instant weight loss but fat, by its nature, cannot dissolve overnight or melt away. Even though we know this, it does not stop us from trying fad diets that promise instant miracles.

These type of diets do not change your eating habits or teach you how to deal with normal eating problems such as social eating, travelling and the yearning for something sweet, salty or fried.

Losing weight fast means you lose predominately water and lean body tissue, not fat. This weight loss is not permanent and soon, when you revert back to your old eating habits, the weight piles on and fat cells swell. To lose ten pounds of fat a week you would have to eat 5,000 less calories a day. A total impossibility!

This sounds depressing and confusing. So how do you do it, especially if you are calorie conscious?

Firstly, you need to understand why you are eating too much, or too much of the wrong types of food. Then you need to aim to achieve your weight loss over a period of time.

If you want to be thinner on the beach this summer, allow a minimum of ten weeks to lose 14lbs (6kgs) of fat. 1lb of fat = 3,500 calories. To lose 1lb of fat a week, you need to reduce your total weekly calorie intake by 3,500 calories or 500 calories a day. Drastic calorie reduction, eating below 1200–1500 calories a day, is dangerous and unhealthy. Your metabolic rate needs a basic 1200–1500 calories a day for your body to simply function. Avoid living off liquid diets or any diet in which your calorie intake is below 1,000 calories a day.

If you are a dietholic what I am asking you to do is to analyse your choice of diet. You could make an appointment to see a dietician or nutritionist. Let them create your own personal diet plan. Have a blood test arranged by your doctor to see if your weight problem and food bingeing is connected to a food allergy.

You are an intelligent human being, so why abuse your body with fad dieting? Even living off brown rice or fruit for weeks on end is a cranky, unbalanced diet. Learn how to analyse a diet before you continue with your dieting, then takes some responsibility for your diet choice.

Answer these questions in relation to your diet

	Yes	No
Do the types of food you eat vary?		
Does your diet allow you to eat food from all food groups, or is it limiting?		
1. Complex carbohydrate – beans, wholegrain bread, potatoes, rice and pasta.		
2. Lean meat – poultry/fish – white, chicken, turkey, tuna (not in oil).		
3. Dairy products – skimmed milk, low-fat yogurts, cheeses and fromage frais.		
4. Plenty of vegetables and fruit of all colours?		
5. Does your diet cater for social occasions and allow you to eat out?		
6. Does your diet consider convenience foods?		
7. Does your diet require you to weigh and measure your food?		
8. Does your diet require you to cook?		
9. Is following your diet time-consuming and fussy?		
10. Does your diet ban all so-called forbidden foods?		
11. Will your diet cater for your sweet tooth?		

The key to success is that the simplest, healthiest diets to follow are those based on healthy eating plans, with the only reductions being in sugars, fats and salt, and allowing all foods in moderation.

Eat To Win

Old habits die hard. You may think it is impossible to change, especially if you are hooked on junk, sweet, high-fat, salty or fried foods.

Can you imagine what it would be like if you could only eat your favourite food and nothing else if you were a junk-food addict? Try it for a few days. Try eating nothing but chips, chocolate or ice-cream. Do not mix the food choice, simply eat one food only. Soon your body and your mind will cry out for a different taste. You are very likely never to want to eat that food again. Go on a junk binge for a few days then stand in front of the best supermarket display of fresh fruit and vegetables. You will find your mouth will be watering, you will be yearning to eat fresh vegetables, salads and fruit – your taste buds will be crying out for real, wholesome foods.

Deny your body something and you will want it, whatever it is. The art of changing your eating habits is to learn to enjoy wholesome food choices and to eat in moderation those so-called forbidden foods. Moderation means not at every meal. If you are a sugar junkie try to restrict yourself to having something sweet only after you have eaten a meal once a day. By using control you are not denying yourself but reducing the desire and slowly re-educating those taste buds.

FOOD CHECK

Fill in the following to see what attitude you have towards food. Once you have filled in each section look through your answers and reflect on them to see where your downfall lies.

Which of the following resembles your eating pattern?

	Yes	No
Three meals a day		
Two meals a day		
You eat nothing all day		
You eat when tired		
You do not eat breakfast		
You feel sleepy around 4pm and eat		
You cannot stop eating bits all the time		
You are always finishing off children's food		
You only eat in the evening		
You eat when you are happy or sad or bored		
You always eat a lot before your period		

Are you addicted to:

	Yes	No
Coffee		
Textured food		
Tea		
Sweet food		
Salt		
Salty food		
Bread		
Wine		
Fried food		
Beer		
Crispy food		
Cigarettes		
Oily food		
Chocolate		

It is time to make changes. Tick off what you can easily cope with changing now and have another go in two weeks time.

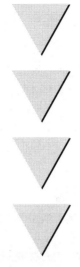

It takes time to adjust to a healthier eating plan. Make what changes you can, however small. Patience is the key – forget the all-or-nothing attitude because trying to completely change overnight never works. Re-educating your tastes and desires is a slow process.

This is one way you can track your progress. For example, the thought of not adding salt to cooked food may seem impossible but within a month it will not be important to you because your taste will have changed.

I CAN:

	Now		2 wks		4 wks	
	Yes	**No**	**Yes**	**No**	**Yes**	**No**
Eat three meals per day or five small meals per day.	▨	▨	▨	▨	▨	▨
Reduce my coffee intake to two cups per day.	▨	▨	▨	▨	▨	▨
Carry a bottle of mineral water around to drink continuously throughout the day.	▨	▨	▨	▨	▨	▨
Drink one glass of wine – not half a bottle.	▨	▨	▨	▨	▨	▨
Stop drinking beer and spirits.	▨	▨	▨	▨	▨	▨
Cut out cakes, pastries, crisps, nuts, sweets and chocolate.	▨	▨	▨	▨	▨	▨
Stop eating ice-cream and croissants.	▨	▨	▨	▨	▨	▨
Stop eating fast food – hamburgers, fish and chips, pizzas, hot dogs, pie and chips.	▨	▨	▨	▨	▨	▨
Stop cooking with salt and adding it to food.	▨	▨	▨	▨	▨	▨
Use salt-reduced soy sauce when cooking.	▨	▨	▨	▨	▨	▨
Stop eating take-aways.	▨	▨	▨	▨	▨	▨
Spoil myself in other ways without eating food for comfort.	▨	▨	▨	▨	▨	▨
Eat a variety of food every day.	▨	▨	▨	▨	▨	▨
I can eat slowly, without distraction or on the run.	▨	▨	▨	▨	▨	▨
I can listen to my body's needs and not make emotional food choices.	▨	▨	▨	▨	▨	▨

I will try and eat more:

	Yes
Apples	▨
Asparagus	▨
Beans	▨
Berries	▨
Bread	▨
Broccoli	▨
Brussel sprouts	▨
Cabbage	▨
Carrots	▨
Cauliflower	▨
Celery	▨
Chicken	▨
Courgettes	▨
Cucumber	▨
Grapes	▨
Leafy salad	▨
Lean meat	▨
Leeks	▨
Melon	▨
Onions	▨
Oranges	▨
Pasta	▨
Peaches	▨
Pineapple	▨
Potatoes	▨
Rice	▨
Seafood	▨
Spinach	▨
Tomatoes	▨
Turkey	▨
White fish	▨

Ticking off what you eat may appear silly but I have had girls tell me in class that they never eat fruit or greens. There is a whole generation of young people who have been brought up on fast foods who never cook for themselves and never experiment with food tastes. Your body is a temple, a shrine, an amazing machine. Give it the best. I am not talking about becoming a brown-rice and bean-sprout freak, I am saying eat real food. Most of my clients have lost weight when they started to eat real foods and planned their meals. When they balanced their food choices they ate a healthy, low-fat selection of foods, allowing for something sweet but junk food and fast food were out.

NUTRITIONAL GUIDELINES

1. Eat slowly. Focus on what you are eating. Avoid distractions, such as TV, that cause you to eat too fast. Savour your meal.

2. Eat three meals or five small meals a day. Do not starve the body until the evening. As your metabolic rate slows down it needs food to burn calories and give your body energy. It is vital to keep your body fuelled and your metabolic rate up. Avoid eating late and heavy meals.

3. Do not make a big deal about food. Thinking about it all day means that you are bored or stressed out. Exercise more and learn to relax.

4. You do not put on weight overnight. Balance your weekly eating if you have social events to attend. Go for the 80–20 percent formula, be sensible 80 percent of the time. Allow 20 percent for social occasions or the odd treat.

5. Reduce your total fat intake by half or more. Try to reduce sugar or sweets, or eliminate them altogether. Limit alcohol. The combination of fat and sugary foods is hard to break down. Add alcohol to a meal and you've created the ideal fat cocktail.

6. Think about your meals. When you eat, think of what your body needs, not what your eyes want. Is your meal nutritionally balanced?

7. Do not substitute a chocolate bar or something sweet for a meal.

8. Remember to drink mineral water every day – at least one and a half litres. Fruit juice is not a substitute, it is a sugar boost without its natural fibre. Fruit juice stimulates hunger by raising your blood sugar which then drops rapidly, stimulating hunger again. Avoid fizzy diet drinks as they have the same effect on your blood sugar. Learn to like water. It is much better than any other drink for boosting your health and your complexion.

9. Carbohydrates do not make you fat. The major part of your meal should consist of a complex carbohydrate, such as wholemeal bread, brown rice, pasta, couscous or potato. Yet, eating too much can make you fat. Excess carbohydrates that are not used in energy will be stored as fat.

Your guide for life

Every day eat:

Liberally All vegetables, wholegrains, whole fruit, wholemeal bread, pasta, rices, buckwheat

Eat moderately Low-fat milk, lean meat, yoghurt, cheese, poultry, fish

Go easy Whole milk, nuts, seeds, sausages, cream, cheese, eggs, fatty meat, butter, game (e.g. duck), margarine, oils, fats, fruit juice

Occasionally All luxury foods, desserts, sweets, alcohol, fats

Base your eating plan on the following food servings which have been taken from the National Food Guide released by the Health Education Authority.

Guidelines are there to help you with the size of your food choices. Many of us know what we should eat but our portion sizes may be too big or small in relation to what our body needs. Everyone has individual serving requirements. It depends on your age, size, sex, activity level and weight. The only way to really know what you should be eating is by having an individual consultation with a dietician. This is why I do not have a diet to go with the programme. I am only giving you guidelines.

What is surprising is that most people do not know how many carbohydrates (e.g. as bread, rice, vegetables, protein and fruit) they can eat. Most people eat too little of these and too much fat from dairy products, animals fats, oils and sugars.

Once you have created the balance with your food choices based on the National Food Guide and increased your activity level, your body composition will change over time and you will drop excess fat.

So let's look at what we should be eating.

I am only using portions related to an active man or woman. The ULBT programme is not about being sedentary. If your activity levels drop due to illness or whatever, be aware of your portion sizes. Reduce them slightly especially the fats and the sugars.

Carbohydrates

Are the best food for energy, fibre and the B vitamins.

Choose complex carbohydrates such as wholemeal bread, grains, potatoes, cereals, pulses and pasta. Avoid refined sugars and flours.

one portion = 1 slice of bread or 1 bread roll

1 (175g/6oz) potato

2 tablespoons cooked rice or pasta

Active women aged 19–49 need to eat seven to ten portions a day.

Active women aged 50–65 plus need to eat six to eight portions a day.

Active men aged 19–49 need to eat ten to eleven portions a day.

Active men aged 50–65 plus need to eat seven to ten portions a day.

Vegetables and Fruit

Are high in essential vitamins, minerals, antioxidants fibre and carbohydrates. These nutrients help improve the body's ability to fight infection, heal and reduce the risk of cancer, high blood pressure and constipation.

Fruits are the best fast energy foods around, which is why so many fitness people eat bananas. Eat as many varied coloured vegetables and fruit, especially vegetables. Steam or stir-fry, avoid boiling the vitamins and minerals away.

1 portion = 2 tablespoons of vegetable

1 piece of fresh fruit

1 small salad fresh

1 small portion of fresh fruit juice 100ml/3½ fl oz

Active men and women aged 19–49 and 50–65 plus should aim to eat a minimum of five portions a day. This could be two servings of fruit and three portions of vegetables.

I do not think you can overeat on vegetables. Sometimes people go overboard on fruit and fruit juice, especially in the summer time. As long as you are active and using up those sugar calories, this will be no problem. It is when you are lazing around that eating masses of fruit can be a problem.

Dairy foods

Milk, cheese and yoghurt supply your body with calcium protein, essential B vitamins, phosphorus and zinc. Essential for maintaining strong bones, hair, healthy teeth and good eyesight. Dairy foods are a vital food source for babies and young children. Maintaining a high calcium intake for the prevention of osteoporosis is vital especially in women over the age of thirty-five.

Go for low-fat milk (adults only), bio-yoghurt and low-fat cheese. Other excellent sources of calcium are tofu, sardines and spinach.

1 serving = 200ml/ ½ pint semi-skimmed milk

40g/1½oz bio-yoghurt, fromage frais, cottage cheese

Active women of all ages need two to three portions a day. Pregnant and breast-feeding women need more. Seek a dietician's advice, and tell them you

exercise on a regular basis.

Active men 15–49 need three portions and active men 50–65 need two to three portions a day.

Meat, Fish, Poultry, Beans

Provides protein for proper muscle development, growth and repair and prevents anaemia.

Protein supplies B vitamins for a healthy nervous system and digestion, minerals, zinc and magnesium for healthy skin, bones and growth. Excess protein is not stored as bulging muscles. Choose low-fat, lean meat, fish, poultry, soya and pulses. Lower the fat intake by grilling or baking.

1 portion = 200g/7oz of cooked pulses

2 eggs (4 a week maximum)

0–70g/2–3oz chicken, lean meat

100–150g/4–5oz white fish only

2tbsp/50g/2oz nuts, peanuts, butter

Active women aged 19–49 need approximately three portions a day.

Active women aged 50–65 plus need approximately two portions a day.

Active men aged 15–65 need approximately three portions a day.

Fats

The word 'fat' creates confusion for most of us. We have the impression that fats are bad for us, but essential fats are necessary for structured compounds in our body such as blood lipids, cell membranes, bile, hormones, vitamin D and natural steroids, and we need fat for sex drive, fertility and a healthy pregnancy. Fats regulate body temperature, synthesize vitamins in the body and are a form of energy. Some essential fatty acids cannot be made by the body and can only be obtained through diet. Fat is the most concentrated source of calories containing about 9 calories per gram, twice as many as protein or carbohyrate. There are three types of fat – saturated, unsaturated and trans fats.

Saturated

These fatty acids are found in butter, cheese, meat, palm and coconut oil – fats that are solid until heated. Saturated fats increase blood cholesterol levels, increasing the risk of coronary heart disease. Butter is a saturated fat so should be avoided by those with a high cholesterol level. I use a small amount of butter instead of margarine as I prefer more natural products.

Unsaturated

These tend to be in liquid forms such as vegetable oils and are divided into polyunsaturates and monosaturates. The body makes its own saturated and monosaturated fat from excess carbohydrates and proteins:

Polyunsaturated fatty acids

Good sources are olive oil, sunflower oil, soya beans, walnuts, rapeseed oil and oily fish. The body cannot make polynsaturated fatty acids which are essential for one's health.

Monosaturates

Good sources are nuts, avocados, seeds, olive oil and rapeseed oil. Use margarines made with olive oil.

Trans fats

These hydrogenated oils – oils made to go hard – are the margarine and fats found in processed foods. Recent research has linked hard margarine to heart disease.

A diet with a low animal fat intake and a high intake of olive oil is thought to lower the risk of heart disease. A high intake of fish oils may protect against cancer of the breast, bowel and pancreas; all of which are associated with high-fat diets and obesity. The message from the experts is clear: reduce your total daily fat intake, especially saturated, trans and hydrogenated fats.

Do

▶ Aim to keep your fat intake to 30 percent of your daily calorie intake. Saturated fat should only form 10 percent of your diet.

▶ Remove all visible fat from your meat.

▶ Choose low-fat or fat-free dairy products.

▶ Create meals from lean proteins, e.g. skinless chicken breast, white fish, tofu, soya.

▶ Steam, stir-fry, grill or bake your food.

▶ Use a light oil spray.

▶ Use margarine made with olive oil.

▶ Use a small amount of butter:

One portion = 1 teaspoon of butter or margarine
1 teaspoon of cooking oil
1 teaspoon of salad dressing
2 teaspoons of low-fat spread

Active women and men need to limit these to once or twice a day.

▶ Balance your diet. If you eat a chocolate bar, make low-fat or no-fat food choices for the rest of the day.

▶ Read all food labels to check the fat and calorie content.

To work out fat percentages, multiply the fat grams given by 30. If the answer exceeds the total amount of calories, the product has over 30 percent fat content. Remember to try and keep within a daily 30 percent fat intake.

Don't

▶ Eat convenience foods, because fats are used as flavour enhancers.

▶ Buy take-aways, as they are full of hidden fats.

Limit sugary and salty foods to once a day or even less for cakes, chocolate, sweets, sausages, paté, sugary cereals and creamy sauces.

Foods that are based on fat or sugar have very few nutrients compared to wholesome foods. Eat them as a treat and restrict your intake for weight loss.

ACTIVE WOMEN SHOULD EAT DAILY:

0
sugar, salty foods, junk - *eat occasionally*
1 2 3
olive oil, sunflower oil - *eat 3 small portions*
1 2 3
meat, beans, fish - *eat 3 portions*
1 2 3
milk, yoghurt - *eat 3 portions*
1 2 3 4 5
vegetables and fruit - *eat 5 portions*
1 2 3 4 5 6 7 8 9 10
rice, bread, pulses, grains - *eat 7–10 portions*

Plan your daily food choices using this nutritional pyramid. Portions are based on the 1994 National Food Guide.

ATTACK THE FAT

1lb of fat = 3,500 calories

Simply switch from high fat-foods to low-fat options and you will reduce your overall fat and calorie intake. Increase your activity and the excess weight will drop off.

Follow these simple rules to reduce your fat intake.

▶ Learn to use a fat substitute such as low-fat fromage frais instead of cream or cream cheese. Follow the American example by using apple sauce, prune purée or concentrated apple juice as a fat and sugar substitute in baking, and reduce the amount of fat and sugar in recipes by 50 percent.

▶ Look on the labels for foods that contain no more than 3g of fat per 100 calories.

▶ Chicken and fish are a healthy option when eaten baked or grilled – it is the sauces that are high in fats. Avoid any sauce using cream or butter, and avoid products coated in breadcrumbs – even if you are grilling the food. Try the Oriental option – grill thin slices of chicken, turkey, beef and fish, and marinate in teriyaki sauce.

▶ Don't snack on savouries such as crisps and salty peanuts, especially when you are drinking. Avoid the peanut bowl in a bar – people do not always wash their hands after visiting the bathroom.

▶ Keep your fat intake to around 30 percent of your total daily food intake. This includes the so-called 'invisible fat' in foods such as cheese, milk and food products in biscuits and cereals.

▶ Go for lean meat (moderately), poultry, fish, seafood and low-fat dairy products.

▶ Avoid lard, dripping, suet, full-cream milk, butter and cheese.

▶ Restrict egg yolks to no more than two per week. Make omelettes with several egg whites and one egg yolk.

Fat Facts

For a healthy body, use a little oil in your food every day: monosaturates (olive oil, hazelnut oil, almond oil, sesame oil), or polyunsaturates (corn oil, sunflower oil, safflower oil, soybean oil, groundnut oil) are valuable food for your body. Use in salad dressing or when cooking a stir-fry.

Using a low-fat substitute does not always work because one has the tendency to eat more because the product states it is low in fat. Ice-cream is the prime example as low in fat does not necessarily mean low in calories. Do not eliminate fat totally from your diet. Fat is essential for body warmth, energy, healthy hormone development and the function of a woman's monthly cycle. It is essential for strong bones, healthy hair, nails and a beautiful complexion.

Only eat lean meat two or three times a week.

Although it may be lean and low in fat, it is still high in saturated fat which is bad for the heart. The solution is to eat more fish.

Low-calorie does not mean low-fat. A ready-made meal may state it is only 300 calories but 50 percent of those calories may come from fat, so read the labels and check the fat grams.

If your energy is low or you are too tired to work-out, avoid grabbing a chocolate bar and then doing a work-out. You are not going to get the results you want. Eat fruit, such as a banana, or have a fresh fruit juice drink for that quick energy boost before working-out.

The combination of sugar and fat is a calorie time bomb, which is why chocaholics have such a hard time managing their weight. For a sweet tooth, try substitutes such as meringue or fruit.

A high-fat diet will make you put on weight because fat is more calorific than carbohydrates and proteins. Each gram of fat you eat produces 9 calories. Each gram of carbohydrates produces 4 calories. Do not become a calorie-counting bore but do read labels and eliminate foods with a high fat content.

Warning – Osteoporosis and diet

Many women avoid dairy products totally to reduce their fat intake and to save on calories. Unfortunately, these women do not realize that a diet high in calcium is vital in preventing the brittle-bone disease osteoporosis. A compromise can avoid health complaints later in life. Drink low-fat skimmed milk and eat low-fat dairy produce such as cottage cheese. Use fat substitutes which supply a requirement of calcium without a high fat content. Other sources of calcium are green vegetables, pulses, oily fish, sardines, nuts and tofu.

MEAL PLANNER

I am not here to write a host of meal planners. There are hundreds of healthy, low-fat recipe books available, but I have enclosed a meal planner guide.

These food choices are easy and quick to prepare so it is possible to always eat a healthy low-fat option.

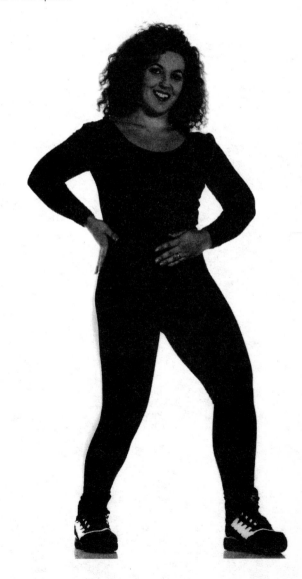

LEISURELY	ULTRA HEALTHY	QUICK	ON THE RUN

Breakfast

LEISURELY	ULTRA HEALTHY	QUICK	ON THE RUN
Fruit juice Boiled egg Wholemeal toast Tea **or** Small bowl muesli (low-sugar variety) with low-fat milk Fruit Juice **or** 2 Weetabix topped with strawberries or banana with low-fat milk Fruit juice	Fresh fruit salad (no melon) Mineral water **or** Stewed apple Banana Tea **or** Low-fat bio-yoghurt with chopped dried apricots. Add 1 tbsp sunflower seeds	Energy drink: ½ pint skimmed milk 1 banana 1 egg white 2 tsp vanilla essence 2 tsp fine bran Liquidize and drink Yoghurt drink: use low-fat bio-yoghurt and fruit of your choice **or** 2 slices wholemeal toast topped with a sugar-free fruit spread. Skimmed milk fresh strawberry shake: 8–10 strawberries 2tbsp plain low-fat bio-yoghurt ¼ litre semi-skimmed milk honey to sweeten (approx 1 tsp)	Mineral water Bananas and grapes **or** 1 bagel Apple or peach **or** Bran muffin Low-fat, shop-bought yoghurt drink Banana

Lunch

LEISURELY	ULTRA HEALTHY	QUICK	ON THE RUN
Large omelette using 1 egg and 4 egg whites stuffed with grilled, chopped mushrooms and ham Serve with salad **or** Grilled or baked white fish topped with fresh basil and tomato. Serve with beans, broccoli and carrots **or** Pancakes made from buckwheat and wholemeal flour. Once cooked add sunflower and sesame seeds. Spread a thin layer of sun-dried tomato paste, ricotta cheese and salad.	2 crispbreads spread with low-fat soft cheese and chives or garlic. Top with 2 sun-dried tomatoes (oil drained). Serve with chopped lettuce **or** Homemade carrot soup 1lb chopped carrots, 1 chopped onion, 1 potato, 2 cloves garlic. Cover with water and add 1 vegetable stock cube. Bring to boil and simmer, liquidize. Dilute with skimmed milk. Season. Add fresh coriander and soy sauce. Serve with fresh bread.	Pitta bread spread thinly with hoummus filled with falafel, lean turkey or chicken and salad (no mayonnaise) **or** Bagel spread with low-fat cream cheese and ready-prepared green salad **or** Grilled ciabatta spread with a thin layer of sun-dried tomato paste, drained tuna and chopped fresh spinach	Low-fat, shop-bought sandwich or baguette with generous filling of chicken or lean ham, tuna or prawn with salad. No mayonnaise or butter **or** Shop-bought baked potato with baked beans or tuna salad **or** Cold chicken leg with vegetable *crudités* **or** Pitta bread with masses of salad and hoummus **or** Ciabatta, sprinkled with 1 tsp of olive oil, masses of sliced tomato on top of thinly-sliced, low-fat mozzarella cheese topped with fresh basil and black pepper **or** Grilled chickenburger, no mayonnaise. Freshly-squeezed orange juice

LEISURELY	ULTRA HEALTHY	QUICK	ON THE RUN

Evening

LEISURELY	ULTRA HEALTHY	QUICK	ON THE RUN
Pasta with steamed broccoli and Parmesan or 2oz low-fat cheese OR Grilled chicken breast with Dijon mustard mixed with fresh lemon juice and sprinkled with black pepper. Serve with steamed French beans and new potatoes tossed in 1 tsp hazelnut oil and fresh parsley.	Baked potato topped with chopped, steamed spinach mixed with garlic fromage frais. Serve with carrots OR Stir-fry finely chopped carrots, cabbage, onion, red pepper, leeks, prawns, soy sauce and garlic in sesame oil. Serve with long-grain rice (brown, wild or basmati)	Instant pizza Spread half a fresh wholemeal stick with tomato purée, slices of lean ham and top with low-fat cheese. Serve with ready-prepared salad from the local supermarket. Dress with an oil and lemon dressing.	You should not eat your evening meal on the run. If you are eating out avoid curry, any meal with a cheese sauce, fried food or vegetables smothered with butter or creamy sauces. OR Go for Italian, Japanese, Mexican or Thai food.

Whatever restaurant you are in, you, as the customer, have the right to ask for low-fat options such as grilled salmon and steamed vegetables.

For the Sweet Tooth

Snack on sweet popcorn
Try: Meringue nest topped with fruit
Frozen low-fat yoghurts
Low-fat lemon mousse
Exotic fruit salad
Mango and raspberries
Kiwi and banana
Baked banana sprinkled with soft brown sugar and lemon juice
Sesame seed pancakes with lemon juice and maple syrup

Drinks

Throughout the day drink mineral water. If your blood sugar is low try freshly-squeezed juice or a low-fat yoghurt drink. Carry small bottles of fresh juice.

THE ULTIMATE LEGS BUMS 'N' TUMS

Food Diary

Most of us think we eat less than we really do. For the first two weeks of the programme monitor your food intake. Do not go for drastic changes in the first week - simply be aware of and note down what you eat.

Keeping a food diary will help you become aware of what foods you are eating and more conscious of your eating habits.

Fill in the blank diary given here for the first week, then carry a note book around. Read up on out-of-control eating (page 35) and see if this helps you to keep to a healthier nutrition plan.

Example

Time	With whom, where and how?	What was eaten?	How much?	How did you feel?
8am	Family Kitchen Standing up	Sugar puffs Full-fat milk	Two bowls (too much)	Out of control

Saturday

Time	With whom, where and how?	What was eaten?	How much?	How did you feel?

Sunday

Time	With whom, where and how?	What was eaten?	How much?	How did you feel?

Monday

Time	With whom, where and how?	What was eaten?	How much?	How did you feel?

Tuesday

Time	With whom, where and how?	What was eaten?	How much?	How did you feel?

Wednesday

Time	With whom, where and how?	What was eaten?	How much?	How did you feel?

Thursday

Time	With whom, where and how?	What was eaten?	How much?	How did you feel?

Friday

Time	With whom, where and how?	What was eaten?	How much?	How did you feel?

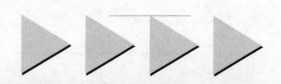

Action Time

▶ **KNOW YOUR MUSCLES** ▶ **HOW TO GET THE MOST FROM YOUR WORK-OUT**
▶ **DO'S AND DON'TS** ▶ **EXERCISE TIPS** ▶ **WARM UP**

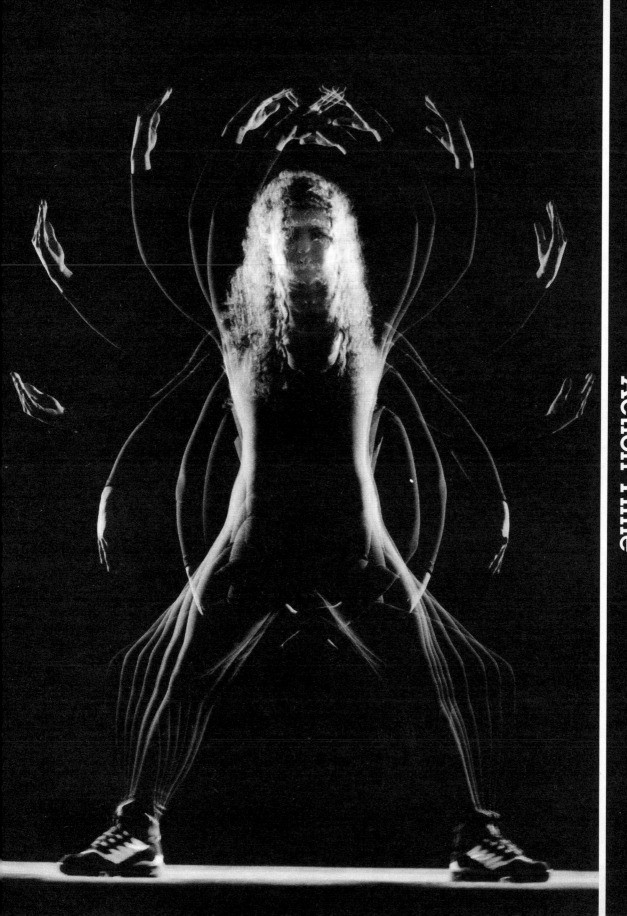

DO NOT JUST EXERCISE WITHOUT AN AIM.

Learn about your muscles and focus your exercises on them for the results you want.

Today there is a lot of exercising material available that can teach us about the structure of our bodies and how we can change them. The exerciser of the Nineties is educated. You should learn where all the major muscles are in your body, their names and what muscles are being targeted during an exercise. One of the main reasons for learning about your body is that mind and body fitness research has shown that if you actually make the mental effort to visualize your muscles working when you exercise, the muscle will respond better and work more efficiently.

Athletes visualize the necessary muscle action to achieve their goals. I visualize all the time, especially when I am presenting new exercises in a masterclass or presenting a stage show. I picture the whole exercise in my mind, including the actual muscular movement. For example, the pelvic floor muscle group is not a muscle with an outward appearance because it is deep inside the body, but when I am demonstrating doing the pelvic floor squeeze (or muscular contraction), I visualize the muscle actually working independently from the rest of my muscles.

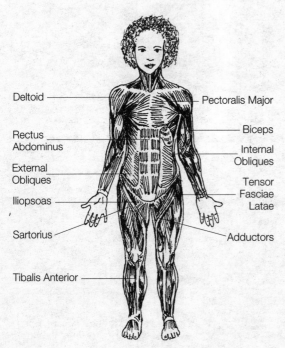

Deltoid
Pectoralis Major
Rectus Abdominus
Biceps
External Obliques
Internal Obliques
Iliopsoas
Tensor Fasciae Latae
Sartorius
Adductors
Tibalis Anterior

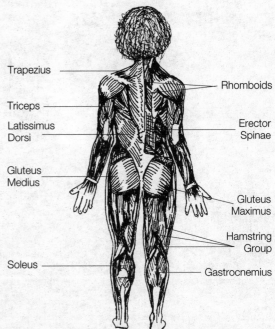

Trapezius
Rhomboids
Triceps
Latissimus Dorsi
Erector Spinae
Gluteus Medius
Gluteus Maximus
Hamstring Group
Soleus
Gastrocnemius

Look at the muscle woman diagrams. Notice all the major muscle groups on the legs, arms, abdominal area and buttocks. These are the muscles you target in your training programme. Seeing them from the inside will help you to relate and focus on them as you work-out.

THESE ARE THE TERMS YOU OFTEN HEAR
FITNESS INSTRUCTORS USE

Muscle Slang

Abbreviation	Muscle Name	Also known as...
Glutes	Gluteus maximus	Bum
	Gluteus medius	
Abs	Rectus abdominus/obliques	Abdominals/tum
Pecs	Pectorals	Chest muscles
Lats	Latissimus dorsi	Back and lower torso
Quads	Quadriceps	Thigh muscles
Hip flexor	Iliopsoas	Front hip area
Adds	Adductors	Inside thigh
Abductors	Tensor Fasciae Latae	Outside thigh

How to get the most from your work-out

Once you have been through the programme, mix and match your routines because muscle thrives on confusion. Beginners should work to the suggested repetitions for each exercise. When this becomes too easy, progress to the whole exercise sequence. In time, after several weeks, you will reach the advanced level.

At first, during the exercises you will be using your body weight and repetitions of the same exercise to overload your muscle work. Overload means that you work the muscle fibre to fatigue. The last few repetitions of the action take a concentrated effort to do as the muscle is tiring from being worked again and again. As you progress and become fitter you will need to challenge your muscles with more resistance. Those used to exercising should add resistance aids to their work-out whenever possible. (The resistance equipment I use in this book is the Forza Body Bar, a weighted bar that also acts as a support, hand weights from 1½ – 2kgs and the Xertube – you should be able to buy the equipment from sports shops, department stores, gyms or chemists.)

All of this equipment is easy to store almost anywhere in the home. One way I motivate myself to exercise at home is by leaving equipment in a prominent place in my bedroom. Most of the time I also have a rebounder and handweights sitting in the corner of my living room, which I use three to four times a week while watching TV.

Before you start, the most essential items for fitness are a good pair of aerobic training shoes – even for body conditioning. Shoes stabilize the foot, especially when you are doing standing leg work.

For women, a good sports bra is essential, whatever size you are. Your outer clothing should be comfortable and allow movement. You should always have a bottle of water nearby to drink throughout the programme. This keeps you hydrated and helps to prevent muscle fatigue.

▶ Change your programme every four to six weeks because your muscles have memory and they will adapt to a programme. In time they will work less efficiently and this can mean up to 25 percent less effort, reducing the amount of calorie expenditure (the amount of calories burnt up during the work-out).

▶ Challenge your aerobic training and intensity. Follow this book's aerobic routine and mix and match the moves. Move stronger and faster for one and a half to two minutes then return to a steady rhythmical pace.

- If you are training aerobically on home equipment such as a bike, rebounder or healthrider, speed up the intensity for two minutes. Do this two to four times during the last fifteen minutes of your aerobic work-out.
- If you decide to do brisk power-walking to burn up those calories, mix up the pace, gently jogging for one minute then walking fast for three minutes. Repeat four or five times during your power-walking session.
- Add on-the-spot fast running. Start with thirty seconds of this and work up to one minute. This outburst is totally anaerobic but you will increase the intensity of the work-out and burn more calories while you keep those muscles alert.

When is the best time to exercise?

There are no firm rules because it really depends on your lifestyle. Research has shown that our metabolism slows down when we sleep. Doing an early evening work-out will increase your metabolic rate for up to fifteen hours, giving you that calorie boost your body needs. However, working out at other times of day still raises your metabolic rate. In ideal circumstances, eat your main meal early, any time from late afternoon to early evening, then work-out for a couple of hours later on (eg 7–8pm). After the work-out, you won't really feel hungry, so have a light snack such as fruit.

Exercise in short bursts

In Chapter 2, Dr James Rippe recommended that the unfit and the beginner would benefit from regular, ten-minute bursts of activity throughout the day adding up to a minimum of thirty minutes. One study of women who did this showed a higher weight loss than those who did a daily thirty-minute work-out session. This is motivational research, as I

know how precious time is. So when time is short do one of the ten-minute work-outs and add in two ten-minute aerobic training sessions every day.

- Some women have an attitude about sweating. Long gone are the days where it was thought that only men sweat and women perspire. In reality you should go for it, working out hard enough to sweat. Sweat keeps the body cool while exercising, and in women it will also alleviate water retention which affects most of us within our monthly hormonal cycles.
- A healthy sweat has been shown to burn more calories and reduce hunger for an hour or so after a work-out. Do not use this as a way not to eat because when you finally do eat, you will be so ravenously hungry that you will probably overeat. Instead, use this natural appetite suppressant to eat in a controlled, sensible manner as soon after a work-out as possible. Carbohydrates fuel our muscles after a work-out in preparation for the next day. Fuelling your muscles within one hour of a work-out is ideal. This is when you should feed yourself with the added benefit of feeling in control!

Exercise do's and don'ts

You will get the most from this programme with the least strain if you follow these guidelines. If you are new to exercise it is advisable to check with your doctor before you begin.

- If you have been totally sedentary start exercising slowly at first. As you go through the programme stick to the beginners level. Doing too much too soon will lead to pain and muscle soreness and you will feel discouraged.
- If you feel tired while exercising, slow down. Do not stop exercising but exercise at a slower, more comfortable pace.
- If you experience any sharp pain or discomfort, tightness in the chest, breathing difficulties or dizziness when exercising, slow down. Then

stop and seek medical advice.

- Never go straight into the routine. Always prepare the body with a warm up.
- Have plenty of water to drink during the work-out. Drink before, during and after the session because you can sweat a great deal during the work-out. Keep your muscles hydrated.
- Do not allow forty-eight hours to pass without exercising. Try to exercise a minimum of three times per week. Aim to do the ULBT programme four to five times a week for real results.
- Do not exercise if you feel unwell.
- If you are inactive for two weeks do not resume the exercise programme where you left off. Work at an easier pace for the first few sessions.
- Do not exercise with an injury. Seek advice then find a way to exercise without using the injured part of your body – if you have a strained ankle, work-out your abs and upper body.
- Do not overtrain. It takes time to get results. If you exhaust your body you will end up injured or ill.
- If you are exercising after a working day on an empty stomach, eat a piece of fruit (such as a banana), or drink some freshly-squeezed orange juice a short while before starting. If you have not eaten since lunch, your energy level will be low due to a drop in your blood-sugar level. To get maximum results from your work-out, you need to give your body fuel. Avoid anything sweet like chocolate.
- Finally, think positive as you work-out. Never think you are a failure, even on an off-day. If you do you may lose your motivation and stop doing the programme. The distractions of life can easily knock you off course, but why let them? You are number one, it is your body, put it first. Simply work-out at an easier level or do the ten-minute plan. Before you start the programme imagine yourself working out. Think how good you will feel afterwards. This is positive thinking.

Warming up

Before beginning the ULBT programme, you need to warm up to prepare your body for the work to come. Preparing the body means increasing your circulation, raising your body temperature and loosening up your joints and all the major muscle groups, stretching and releasing tension from daily stress or poor posture. For example, sitting at a desk all day will weaken your abdominal postural muscles. The warm up is also a time for your mind to focus on the body.

Work-out preparation

- Have a mirror nearby to check your body alignment.
- Take the phone off the hook.
- Tell your family or partner that this is your time, they need to either leave you alone or join in.
- Have mineral water nearby to sip whenever you want.
- If possible, open the windows for fresh air.

For the work-out you will need:

- A broom handle or chair – to be used as a body bar for support, and it also doubles up as an 8lb weight.
- Keep a mat or folded towel ready on the floor.

If you are at an advanced level and you want to use resistance equipment, such as a body bar, light 3–5lb weights in the conditioning sections, tubes or bands, have these ready to use after the warm up.

How hard should you work?

For your muscles to strengthen and tone you need to take the muscle to fatigue. By repeating actions you will create an overload working against your body weight or by using some form of resistance, such as weights or resistance bands.

You need to work the muscle group until it fatigues. *Note:* this must not be sharp pain.

How many repetitions should you do?

The amount of repetitions can vary. You need to repeat the exercise so that you feel the muscle tire without losing your alignment or muscle action. You may find you need to do more repetitions than stated, but beginners should be warned; do not get carried away by doing too much as you can end up feeling extremely sore, especially if your muscles have never exercised. With each exercise or combination I have given guidelines, whether you are a beginner or advanced.

Body check

How conscious are you of your posture? Being aware of your posture enables you to align your body correctly as you work-out. Poor alignment and uncontrolled movements can lead to injury. Correcting poor postural habits does not happen overnight. Muscle strength and flexibility improves gradually. If you continually do a body check as you work-out, you will soon develop good exercise alignment.

LET'S GET STARTED

The time is now yours. Stand tall, feet slightly wider than your hips, chest lifted, shoulders relaxed, tummy pulled in with your tailbone tucked under. Feel your spine lengthen.

Breathe deeply, consciously inhaling through your nose and allowing your chest to lift and your abdominals to expand. Exhale, contracting your abdominals allowing your chest to lower. Focus on this deep breathing for thirty seconds (most of us are shallow breathers in everyday life). Deep breathing takes more oxygen through the blood to the muscles. A better oxygen intake will give the muscles energy for the workload to come.

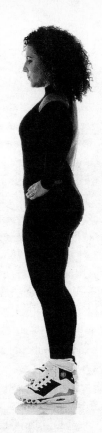

Warm up preparation

Muscles targeted: all the major muscle groups

Start by releasing upper-body tension with a ten-second hold. Clasp your hands, look down and allow your upper back to stretch out, rounding your shoulders. Keep your abdominals contracted, knees bent and tailbone tucked under. Exhale on the stretch, hold for ten seconds.

Now into knee bends and arm raises. Start with your legs wide, knees in line with your heels, tailbone down,

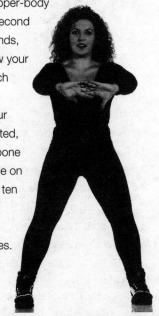

abdominals contracted. Cross your hands in front of your waist and scoop them out and up into a wide arm reach above your head. Lengthen your body as you lift then return to starting position. Exhale as you lift up. Repeat four times. Close your eyes and focus on your deep breathing. Circle your hips to release your lower back, keeping your abdominals contracted. Circle four to the left then four to the right.

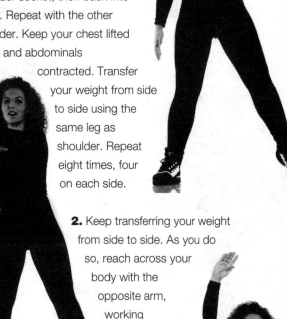

Sequence 1 Warm Up
Shoulder rolls
Muscles targeted: deltoids, trapezius, pectorals, rhomboids

1. Alternating shoulder rolls: Lifting one shoulder roll it forward, up towards your ear, around the shoulder socket, then back into place. Repeat with the other shoulder. Keep your chest lifted and abdominals contracted. Transfer your weight from side to side using the same leg as shoulder. Repeat eight times, four on each side.

2. Keep transferring your weight from side to side. As you do so, reach across your body with the opposite arm, working rhythmically. Keep your chest lifted. Repeat eight times, alternating sides.

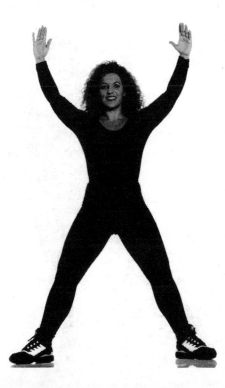

3. Follow on with single-arm sky reaches, reaching across the body and lifting the arms higher. Alternate the arms. Keep your spine lengthened and your abdominals pulled in. Repeat eight times.

Repeat the sequence three times, working rhythmically throughout.

Sequence 2 Warm Up

Marching on the spot

Muscles targeted: quadriceps, hamstrings

1. March on the spot, pumping the arms for sixteen counts.

2. Stand with your feet hip-width apart, abdominals pulled in and tailbone down, ready for hamstring curls. Curl back one leg as if you are trying to kick yourself. Keep your chest lifted. As you do this, curl and pump your arms in time with your legs, alternating the legs. Repeat eight times for both legs.

3. March on the spot for another sixteen counts, then progress to alternating knee lifts, taking your opposite hand to your knees. Keep your body tall, and do not bend your waist.

Repeat the sequence twice.

Warm Up Sequence 3

Squat and side leg lift

Muscles targeted: quadriceps, abductors, adductors

1. Start with a half-parallel squat. The abdominals are contracted, the knees and feet are in line, the tailbone is down. Squat down, then transfer your weight to your right leg.

2. Extend the left leg to the side in a low lift. Bring the leg back to a centre squat and repeat on the other leg. Repeat eight times alternating the legs.

3. Then march briskly on the spot keeping your body lengthened for one minute. Repeat sequence three times. You will need to warm up the body for at least eight minutes before moving into the programme, so repeat the entire warm up four times.

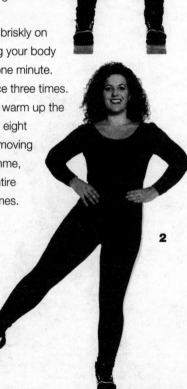

1

2

Stretch Time

Hamstring stretch

Muscles targeted: hamstrings, gluteals

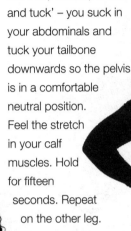

1. Bend your supporting leg. Ease your tailbone back and flex the foot of your extended leg. Avoid locking the knee on the extended leg. With your chest lifted and your abdominals contracted, place your hands on the bent thigh to support your weight. Hold the stretch for fifteen seconds. Repeat on the other leg.

Front of thigh stretch

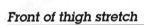

Muscles targeted: quadriceps

2. Use a chair for support, if you find it difficult to hold this position. Standing on one leg, with the abdominals pulled in, bend your knee and lift the other heel behind you, holding on to the ankle with your hand. Keep your body upright, the standing knee soft and aligned with the stretched leg. Aim to feel the stretch on the front of the thigh, not at the knee. Hold for fifteen seconds. Repeat on the other leg.

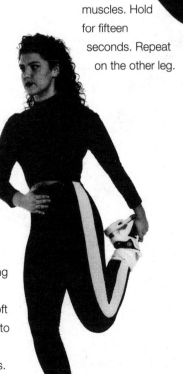

Calf stretch

Muscles targeted: soleus, gastrocnemius

3. Step one leg forward and transfer your weight forward on to it. With your legs close together and bending both knees slightly, press your heels down to the floor. Keep your spine lengthened, your abdominals contracted and your tailbone down. I call this posture position 'suck and tuck' – you suck in your abdominals and tuck your tailbone downwards so the pelvis is in a comfortable neutral position. Feel the stretch in your calf muscles. Hold for fifteen seconds. Repeat on the other leg.

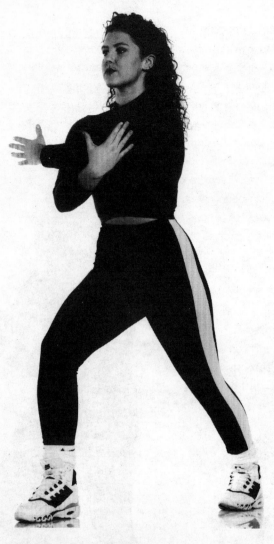

Inner thigh stretch

Muscles targeted: *adductors*

5. Stand tall, contracting your abdominals. Turn the right foot out slightly. Rotate your left leg from the hip and step it away from the body. Bend the left knee, keeping it in line with or behind the ankle, not in front and transfer your weight to the left leg. Feel the stretch along the left inner thigh and the groin area. Stretch and hold for fifteen seconds. Transfer your weight and stretch the other leg.

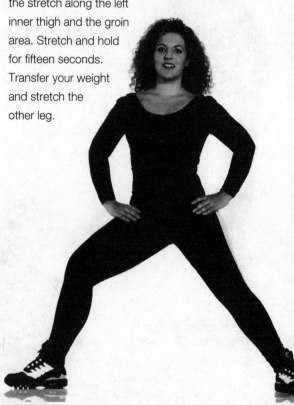

Calf and upper-body stretch

Muscles targeted: *soleus, gastrocnemius, deltoids, rhomboids*

4. Transfer the left leg behind you. With your abdominals contracted, tailbone down, knees and feet in line, bend your right knee, keeping it aligned with the heel. Focus on pressing the back heel down. Feel the calf stretch. Reach across your body with your left arm. Use your right arm to pull it in close to your chest. Feel tension on the outside of the left arm and shoulder. Hold both stretches for fifteen seconds. Exhale as you stretch. Repeat with the right side.

Upper-body stretch

Muscles targeted: rhomboids, latissimus dorsi, erector spinae, deltoids

6. With your legs slightly apart, bend your knees and clasp your hands in front of your chest, palms facing outwards. Pull your hands forward, rounding your back. Focus on rounding the back, and hold for eight seconds. Keep the tailbone down and chest lifted.

Chest stretch

Muscles targeted: pectorals

7. Take the arms back and stretch out the chest to ease the pectoral muscles. Avoid locking the elbows or arching the lower back. Keep the tailbone down and chest lifted as you stretch. Hold for fifteen seconds.

Now you are ready to put those muscles into aerobic action in the next chapter.

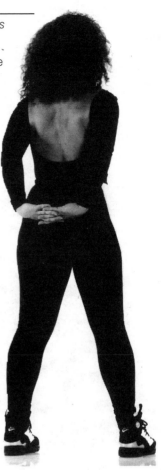

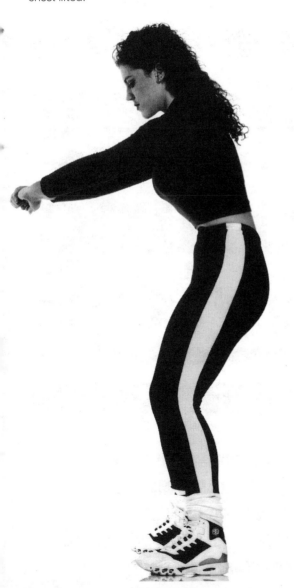

Aerobics
Fat-burning
Exercise

▶ **THE ONLY EXERCISE THAT USES OXYGEN AND GLYCOGEN FOR ENERGY** ▶ **THE ONLY EXERCISE THAT CAN STIMULATE YOUR METABOLIC RATE** ▶ **THE ONLY EXERCISE THAT CAN IMPROVE YOUR CIRCULATION AND LOWER YOUR HEART RATE** ▶ **THE ONLY EXERCISE THAT HELPS PROTECT YOU FROM HEART DISEASE**

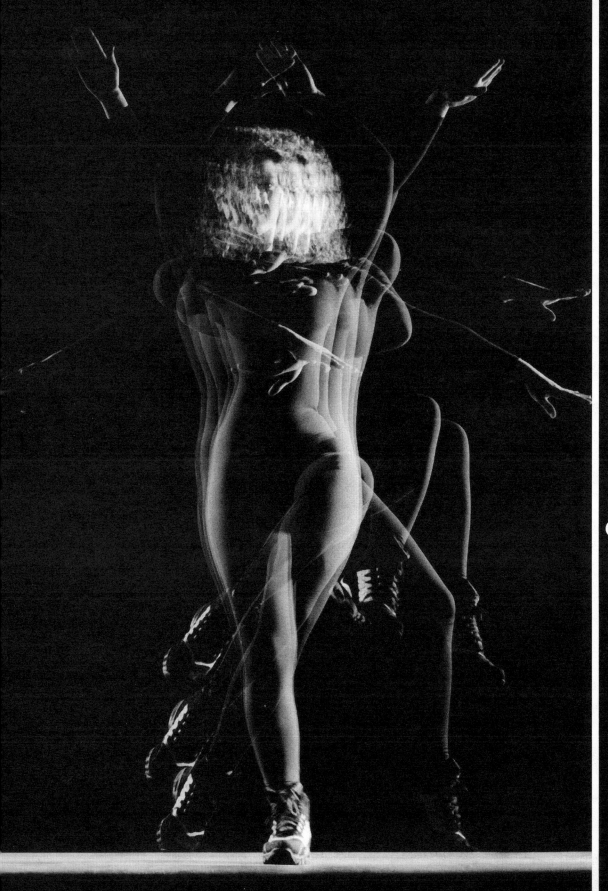

Aerobics Fat-burning Exercise

Why aerobics?

Aerobic exercise is the key that helps you to lose weight and maintain weight loss. Regular aerobic exercise helps to lower the risk of heart disease by strengthening your heart and lungs so that they will become more efficient at transporting blood around your body and utilizing oxygen. A stronger heart means that it does not have to work as hard pumping blood through your body. It beats less. A stronger heart allows you to cope with everyday activities with less stress.

Through regular aerobic exercise, the body uses fat stores as fuel for energy, leaving the lean muscle tissue. Remember that dieting alone eats into the body's lean muscle tissue. You do not want this to happen. It is the fat you want to lose. You can only do this by combining sensible eating with regular aerobic exercise, because aerobics will increase your metabolic rate by increasing your metabolism. This means that you are increasing the rate of energy burnt during and after exercise. This helps to decrease body fat. Aerobic exercise does not just benefit your heart and lungs, it also reduces the risk of arteriosclerosis by decreasing your blood-cholesterol level.

Aerobic exercise alleviates mild cases of hypertension by lowering blood pressure, creating energy so that you can cope with life. It releases endorphins, naturally occurring chemicals in your body that make you feel good, creating a natural high. It is a great way to release stress.

How often and how hard do I need to exercise?

To gain the benefits of aerobic training you have to exercise aerobically three to five times a week at the right training level for you. The training level or exercise intensity is referred to as the target heart rate (THR).

For efficient fat-burning, depending on your level of fitness, you need to exercise from 60–85 percent of your THR. Your target heart range is 60–85 percent of your maximum heart rate or how many beats per minute your heart is working when exercising.

How to find your THR

To find this, subtract your age from 220, this will give you your maximal heart rate.
Take the example of a 30 year old
220 – 30 = 190
190 x 60 percent = 114
190 x 85 percent = 161.50
the THR is 114 or 161.5 per minute for efficient fat-burning.

To check your work-out is of fat-burning intensity, you need to take your pulse during the aerobic exercise session and immediately afterwards. You can take your pulse at the wrist or at the side of the throat. Feel the pulse with your index finger, count it for ten seconds and then multiply the pulse rate by six, or you can take your pulse for six seconds and multiply by the amount by ten. The end figure will tell you how hard your heart is working per minute.

It takes a lot of practice to be accurate. The best option is to invest in a Polar Monitor.

Use the chart over the page to check your THR range.

Target Heart Rate Training Range

Locate your age and level of fitness.

Heart rate should be taken during exercise or immediately after exercise.

AGE	BEGINNER LEVEL		INTERMEDIATE LEVEL		ADVANCED LEVEL	
	(four to six weeks)		(four to six weeks)		(maintenance)	
	Beats per minute	Beats per 10 seconds	Beats per minute	Beats per 10 seconds	Beats per minute	Beats per 10 seconds
19 and under	120–140	20–24	138–155	23–25	150–174	25–29
20 to 24	120–140	20–24	138–155	23–25	144–174	24–29
25 to 29	115–137	18–22	135–152	22–25	144–166	24–29
30 to 34	110–133	18–22	131–147	21–24	138–162	23–27
35 to 39	110–130	18–21	128–142	21–23	136–160	22–26
40 to 44	96–126	16–21	124–139	20–23	128–151	21–25
45 to 49	96–123	16–20	121–135	20–22	126–146	21–25
50 to 54	90–119	15–19	117–132	19–22	120–142	20–23
55 to 59	90–116	15–19	114–130	19–21	110–139	18–23
60 and older	90–112	15–18	110–127	18–21	100–134	16–22

The chart is the courtesy of The International Exercise for Life Institute (US).

You can exercise aerobically in many ways. From aerobic dance, step, funk to fast walking, cycling, jogging, rowing, cross-country, skiing and on cardiovascular equipment such as a stair master or a stationary bike.

Exercise equipment

If you choose to invest in home cardiovascular (aerobic training) exercise equipment, have a good look around before making your purchase. The home exercise market is very competitive. Depending on your budget you can buy anything from a step machine to a treadmill. My personal favourite is the rebounder (mini-trampoline) and, new to this country, the HealthRider. The HealthRider works every major muscle group in your body during the aerobic work-out and is impact-free on the joints. It is ideal for all ages to use.

Both are reasonably priced but they are also multi-functional. All the family can use them from my four-year-old daughter bouncing away on the rebounder, to my oldest daughter using the HealthRider. Investing in equipment is making a commitment to a fitter lifestyle. If necessary you can buy equipment that you can easily move out of sight.

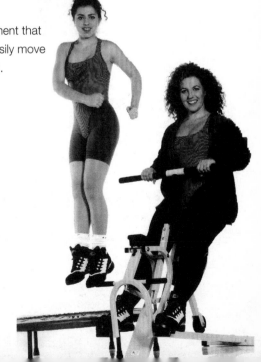

Variety is the spice of life. It is also the lifelong way to aerobic fat-burning success.

As long as you enjoy whatever form of aerobic exercise you choose, you will be able to work long enough for an aerobic training level, three to five times a week. I have illustrated basic aerobic dance moves and a routine to follow, but you may want to invest in home exercise equipment or go power-walking or cycling.

For the best result in maintaining your programme, I suggest you mix your training. Depending on how you feel, you may want to exercise in the privacy of your home, or you may want fresh air and prefer being outside. Whatever you choose to do make sure you add a minimum of three aerobic points to your weekly monitoring chart. 1 point is equal to one twenty-minute session of aerobic activity.

A great motivation tip is to put up an aerobic point chart on the fridge door for the whole household to mark up every twenty-minute aerobic session they do in a week. It will also keep your eating in check.

1 point = twenty minutes of aerobic exercise
2 points = twenty minutes of aerobics plus twenty-five minutes of ULBT

Add an extra 1 point for every ten minutes of extra aerobics you do.

Try to achieve a minimum of 6 points a week. It could be three sessions of twenty-minute aerobics or twenty-five minutes of ULBT.

Calories in calories out, that is what aerobic activity is all about.   ·

The chart shows you the average calories used in exercise, not just aerobic but most forms of exercise. The calorie figures have been based on a person weighing 140lb/63kg.

Average calories used during exercise

Light – 4 Calories per minute
Walking, slow; Gardening, light; Cycling, light ; Body toning; Golf, social; Tennis, doubles; Housework, light; Rebounding, light; Tenpin bowling; Table tennis, social; Horse riding; Ice-skating; Roller-skating/roller-blading; Skate-boarding

Moderate – 7 Calories per minute
Walking, brisk; Aerobics, light; Cycling, moderate; Swimming; Weight-training, light; Tennis, singles; Racketball, beginners; Rebounding, moderate; Football; Basketball; Baseball; Walking, downstairs; Skiing (downhill); Square dancing; Dancing

Heavy – 10 Calories per minute
Jogging; Running; Aerobics, advanced; Swimming, strenuous; Swimming, training; Weight-training, heavy; Wrestling; Judo; Skipping; Racketball, advanced; Football, training; Basketball (pro); Climbing stairs; Skiing (cross-country); Dancing, strenuous

(© The International Exercise for Life Institute (US))

Notes

1. The above figures are for a 140-lb/63-kg person. Add or subtract 10 percent of the calories for each 14lbs above or below 140lb/63kg. The heavier the person, the more energy is expended.

2. Only those sports or activities that are sustained over a period of time (such as running) qualify for heavy exercise. Stop/start sports such as tennis are moderate on average.

Now you have considered this you can assess your lifestyle and set yourself goals. Let's see what activity changes you could make.

Half an hour of brisk walking at lunch time is 210 calories. Five days a week, total = 1,050 calories.

Add four sessions of ULBT a week, using up approximately twenty minutes of aerobics and twenty-five minutes of conditioning, and the total = 960 calories.

You may then go out dancing every weekend for three hours.

It may be clubbing or line dancing, you are simply being active and having fun. Fun = 600 calories.

You also cycle for an hour at the weekend = 420 calories.

Then you blitz the house, two hours of hard housework = 480 calories. Bonus activities you made time for: you managed a half hour moderate swim = 210 calories and a game of tennis for an hour = 410 calories.

Total calories expended:

1,050	=	five days lunch time walks
960	=	four sessions of ULBT
600	=	one night out dancing
420	=	an hour of cycling
210	=	half an hour of swimming
410	=	one hour tennis game
4,230		

This is only a start. As you get fitter you will work-out harder and burn more calories.

By being active all week you have created a calorie demand of 4,230 on your body. Remember 1lb of fat is 3,500 calories. You have also speeded up your metabolic rate so you are using extra calories at rest, plus you have lowered your fat intake by 500 calories a day by cutting out chocolate and biscuits, switching to low-fat foods and grilling, baking or stir-frying your food.

You have lowered your calorie intake by a minimum of 500 calories but you have created extra demands on your body of 4,350 activity calories, a total of 4,850.

You will lose 1lb – 2lb of body fat which is what you want. Any other weight loss is water weight. Losing 1lb – 2lb of weight is the safest, most permanent weight loss at which to aim.

I do not want you to count calories but to become aware of what you are doing in your lifestyle. Any food that is more than your body can use up in activity and through basic maintenance will end up as fat. By eating wisely, not starving yourself, and by making good food choices you use up more calories than you have eaten and you will lose fat!

Aerobic work-out tips

1. Monitor how hard you are working by taking your pulse or doing the talk test, during and immediately after the work-out.
2. Do not exercise in bare feet, invest in a good pair of aerobic shoes.
3. Have water nearby to sip during the work-out.
4. When you are exercising at home make space to move, at least four steps forward, backward and side-to-side.
5. Work-out dynamically by moving continuously for twenty to thirty minutes.
6. Select four to six tracks of motivating, upbeat music to play as you work-out.

Before you start

Remember you have to warm up the body for a minimum of eight minutes before you do any form of aerobic activity.

When you exercise do not work-out too fast or too hard, increase the pace of the aerobics from marching into a jog, pacing it up gradually after a few minutes. Always check how you are feeling throughout your work-out. Your breathing should be fairly laboured, but you should have enough breath to carry on a light conversation. By doing this during the work-out it will insure you are working within your proper training zone.

At the end of the session gradually pace down and then stretch out. Do the stretches on pages 116 -120 for the cool down. If you are new to exercise start slowly and progress gradually. The more often you work-out the easier it will get.

You will notice a significant improvement in your fitness level within six to eight weeks if you work-out three to five times a week.

AEROBIC MOVES

When exercising be aware of your aerobic alignment throughout the work-out. Be conscious of keeping your body lifted, the spine long and the abdominal muscles contracted to support the back. Make sure you do not work-out on your toes by placing the whole foot down from toe to heel during the work-out. Locking or snapping your joints as you work-out can cause harm to the joint. Keep your movements dynamic but controlled, do not snap back the knees or elbows.

Grapevine
(Four-count move)

This is the most common aerobic step in the world. Begin by standing with your feet together. Step to the right side, leading with the right foot. Your left foot follows stepping behind your right foot. You will then step to your right again with the right leg, the left foot follows, and you then step together. Think step wide, cross behind, wide, together. Repeat the Grapevine to the left.

Step touch (not illustrated)
(Two-count move)

Begin by standing with your feet together, then your left foot steps to the left and your right foot follows, tapping down next to the left. Repeat to the right with the right foot leading, the left foot tapping down.

Squat 'n' clap
(Four-count move)

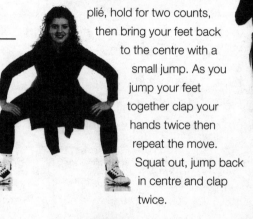

Begin by standing with your feet together. Take your left leg out to the side, bend both knees in a plié, hold for two counts, then bring your feet back to the centre with a small jump. As you jump your feet together clap your hands twice then repeat the move. Squat out, jump back in centre and clap twice.

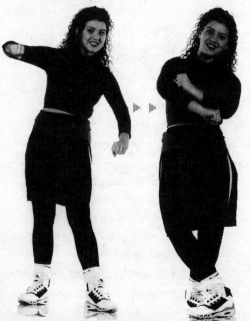

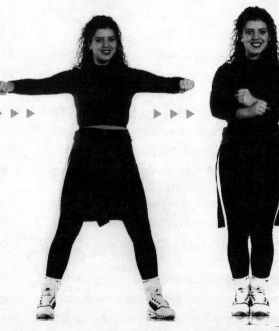

Mambo

(Four-count move)

Go for the Latin feel here. Begin by standing with your feet together. Step forward diagonally with your left leg crossing your right. Allow your hips to sway forward with the move, transferring your weight back. Step back on to your right foot allowing your hips to sway back. Bringing your left foot back to the centre, your feet are now together. Allow your arms to move forward with the movement. Now repeat the mambo on the other side.

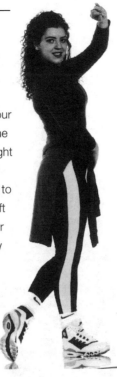

Jumping Jack (not illustrated)

(Two-count move)

Begin with your feet together. Jump your feet apart, with your legs turned out from the hips, knees and feet aligned. Bend your knees on landing, place your heels on the floor, then jump your feet back together again.

Alternating knee lift

(Four-count move)

Begin with your feet together. Step your right leg forward and lift your left knee up towards your right hand. Keep the knee lower then hip level and bring your ankle up to meet your right hand. Do not bend your back, and keep the abdominals contracted. Place the foot down and repeat on the opposite leg.

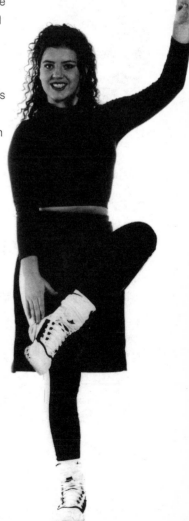

Pivot turn

(Four-count move)

Begin by standing with your feet together. Your left foot remains on the spot. Your right foot steps forward and around, turning your body towards the left, pivoting on the ball of the foot. Take three steps on three counts to pivot around until you are facing forward again.

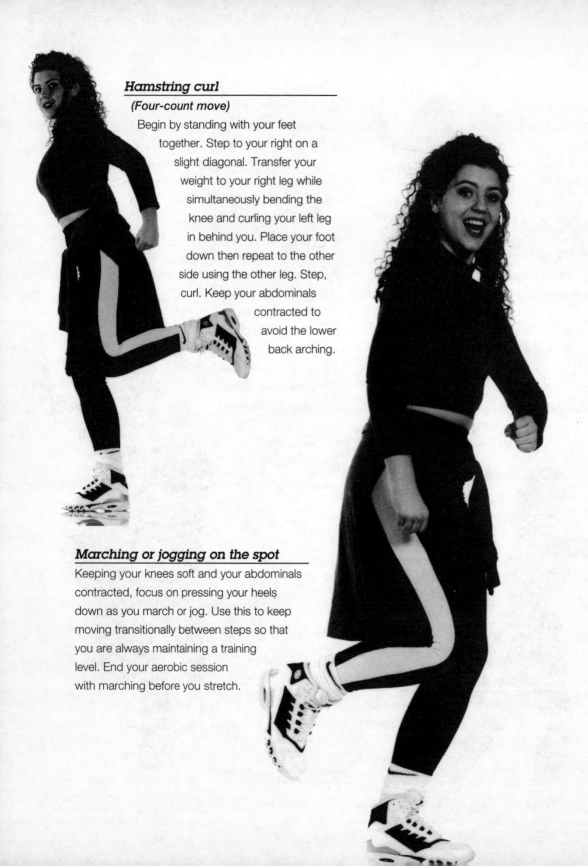

Hamstring curl

(Four-count move)

Begin by standing with your feet together. Step to your right on a slight diagonal. Transfer your weight to your right leg while simultaneously bending the knee and curling your left leg in behind you. Place your foot down then repeat to the other side using the other leg. Step, curl. Keep your abdominals contracted to avoid the lower back arching.

Marching or jogging on the spot

Keeping your knees soft and your abdominals contracted, focus on pressing your heels down as you march or jog. Use this to keep moving transitionally between steps so that you are always maintaining a training level. End your aerobic session with marching before you stretch.

Do this aerobic routine to your chosen music. It needs to be upbeat. As you do the routine, increase the effort after a few minutes marching.

Grapevine left. March on the spot for four counts.
Grapevine left. Squat and clap. Grapevine right.
Squat and clap. March forwards for three counts, toe tap on four.
March backwards for three counts, tap behind on four.
Squat and clap.
Mambo left for two counts, then leading with your right foot, do three quick steps.
Mambo to your right for two counts, then leading with your left foot do three quick steps.
Grapevine left. Squat and clap.
March forward four counts, mambo left.
Mambo right and three quick steps.
March back four counts.
Jumping jack twice on the spot.
Grapevine left. Jumping jack twice.
Grapevine right.
Pivot turn to the right, using the left foot as the pivot.
Grapevine left, pivot turn to the left.
Mambo left and three quick steps.
Grapevine right.
Pivot turn and mambo right and three quick steps.
March on the spot for six counts.
Then change rhythm to:
Step touch left, step touch right. Repeat eight times.
Knee lift right, knee lift left, repeat eight times.
Grapevine left. Squat and clap.
Grapevine right. Squat and clap.
March or jog forwards for two counts, jumping jack for two counts and repeat twice.
Pivot turn, outward left leg squat, and clap.
Grapevine right. Squat and clap.
Grapevine left. Squat and clap.
Jog forwards for two counts, jumping jack for two counts and repeat twice.
Pivot turn outwards on right leg.

Squat and clap twice.
Squat and clap twice.
Hamstring curl left, hamstring curl right.
Repeat eight times.
Step touch left, step touch right. Repeat eight times.
March down sixteen counts.

However you mix and match your steps have fun and make sure you notch up three to four aerobic points a week. Remember to check how hard you are working-out during and immediately after the work-out, using the talk test or pulse monitoring.

After your twenty-minutes aerobic session, stretch out your leg muscles ready for the conditioning section to come. Stretch the front of thigh, the quads, the back of the leg, the calves and hamstring, the inner thighs and the adductor muscles. They are the same stretches you did in the warm up on pages 62-7.

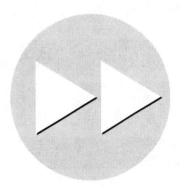

Legs

SHAPE THOSE MUSCLES

▶ **DO IT RIGHT** ▶ **STANDING EXERCISES**
▶ **SMOOTH, CONTROLLED MUSCLE ACTION** ▶ **OVERLOAD THE**
MUSCLE WORK USING YOUR BODY WEIGHT

Legs

DO IT RIGHT

Before you start toning your muscles, you need to learn a few basics about exercising. Doing it wrong can lead to muscular strain and injury. If you are used to exercising you may not be interested in this section but it is always a good idea to do a body check.

Think of your body alignment when you exercise.

Do it right: Wide Plié

Muscles targeted: abductors, quadriceps, gluteals, adductors

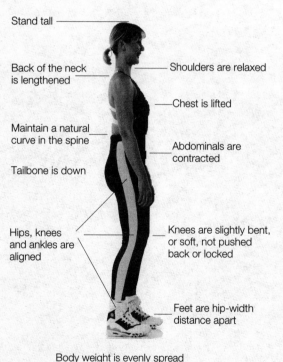

Stand tall

Back of the neck is lengthened

Shoulders are relaxed

Chest is lifted

Maintain a natural curve in the spine

Abdominals are contracted

Tailbone is down

Hips, knees and ankles are aligned

Knees are slightly bent, or soft, not pushed back or locked

Feet are hip-width distance apart

Body weight is evenly spread

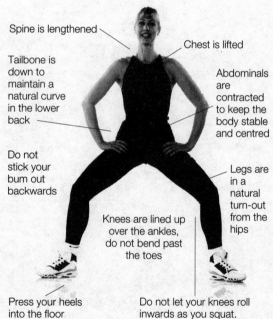

Spine is lengthened

Chest is lifted

Tailbone is down to maintain a natural curve in the lower back

Abdominals are contracted to keep the body stable and centred

Do not stick your bum out backwards

Legs are in a natural turn-out from the hips

Knees are lined up over the ankles, do not bend past the toes

Press your heels into the floor

Do not let your knees roll inwards as you squat.

Stand with your legs turned out slightly wider than hips.

It takes time to feel comfortable and natural with the correct exercise posture. Most teachers and dancers stand like this. It will become second nature to you if you work at it.

As you lower your body, contract the abdominals and focus on pressing downwards into your thighs. As you lift, focus on contracting or squeezing the adductors, gluteals and quadriceps upwards as you move.

Do it right: Lunges

Muscles targeted: *quadriceps, gluteals, hamstrings*

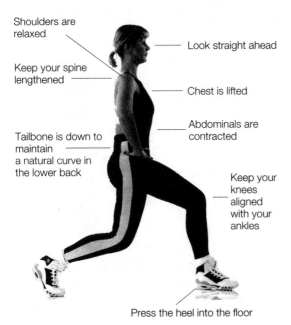

Shoulders are relaxed

Look straight ahead

Keep your spine lengthened

Chest is lifted

Abdominals are contracted

Tailbone is down to maintain a natural curve in the lower back

Keep your knees aligned with your ankles

Press the heel into the floor

Wrong

Do not lunge so deeply that your back knee touches the floor or you feel strain or knee pain. Never bend beyond the toes.

Wrong

Do not step so far forwards or backwards that you cannot return to standing without losing your alignment or creating pressure on the lower back.

Lunges are a great exercise for toning the legs and the bum. To avoid knee and lower-back strain it is essential that you focus on getting it right. In an exercise you can do a stationary lunge, a forward or a backward lunge. Even a travelling lunge, as with all types of lunging, you target the same muscle groups and need to apply all of the safety training tips.

Do it right: Side Leg Raises

Muscles targeted: *abductors, gluteals, medius, minimus, tensor fasciae*

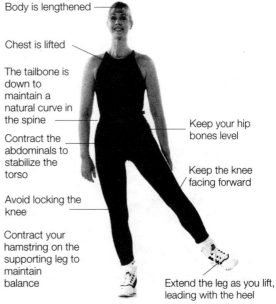

Body is lengthened

Chest is lifted

The tailbone is down to maintain a natural curve in the spine

Keep your hip bones level

Contract the abdominals to stabilize the torso

Keep the knee facing forward

Avoid locking the knee

Contract your hamstring on the supporting leg to maintain balance

Extend the leg as you lift, leading with the heel

Avoid lifting so high that you lose your alignment in the standing leg (for example, the hip will jut out).

You can vary how you target the muscles by rotating the leg outwards from the hip. As you lift the leg away from your body, focus on pressing outwards. When you bring the leg inwards, focus on squeezing the inner thighs together.

Squats

Muscles targeted: *quadriceps, gluteals, hamstrings, adductors*

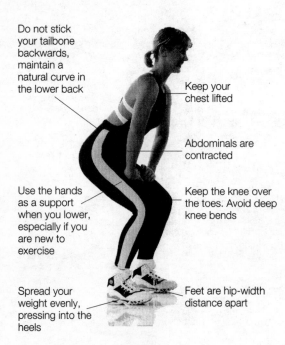

Do not stick your tailbone backwards, maintain a natural curve in the lower back

Keep your chest lifted

Abdominals are contracted

Use the hands as a support when you lower, especially if you are new to exercise

Keep the knee over the toes. Avoid deep knee bends

Spread your weight evenly, pressing into the heels

Feet are hip-width distance apart

Keep the action smooth and controlled as you lower into a squat. You can overload your muscle work by adding resistance equipment.

There is no benefit in doing a deep squat, you are not a power-lifter. Squatting too deeply causes strain on the knees and the lower back.

Focus on pressing downwards through your backside as you lower, then squeeze the inner thighs together as you rise to standing.

SHAPE THOSE MUSCLES

Standing Leg Combo

Muscles targeted: *abductors, gluteals, hamstring, adductors, quadriceps, iliopsoas*

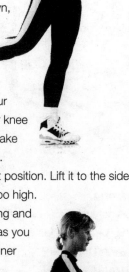

Side leg squeeze

1. Standing tall, using a chair or pole for support, the tailbone is lengthened down, the spine is long, the abdominals are contracted and the chest is lifted.
Transfer your weight to your standing leg. Keeping your knee forward and slightly bent, take your left leg out to the side.
Maintain it in a slightly bent position. Lift it to the side then lower, avoid lifting it too high.
Repeat eight times, pressing and squeezing the outer thigh as you lift up and squeezing the inner thigh as you lower.

Leg extension and curl

2. Maintain your posture. Extend the right leg behind you squeezing into the glute muscles, lifting only a few centimetres off the floor. Lift and squeeze.
Repeat eight times.

5. Lift the right leg up and move it across in front of you, gripping your inside thighs and squeezing your buttocks as you do this. Take it back out to the side and repeat eight times.

Point and extend

6a. Finally, move your right foot back down towards the floor. Touch your toe to the floor. **b.** Lift and extend the leg in front of you.

Keep your abdominals contracted, hips stationary and avoid lifting the leg above hip level. Lift and lower eight times.

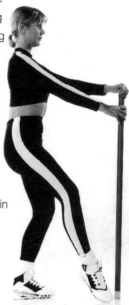

6a.

Repeat the whole sequence on the left leg.
Beginners: aim to do two repetitions, work gradually through the sequence.
Advanced: aim for four sets.

Body check

Maintain your exercise posture throughout the sequence by contracting your abdominals and maintaining a natural curve in the spine. Shake out any muscular discomfort during the sequence.

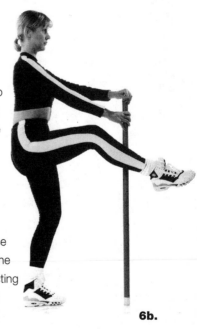

6b.

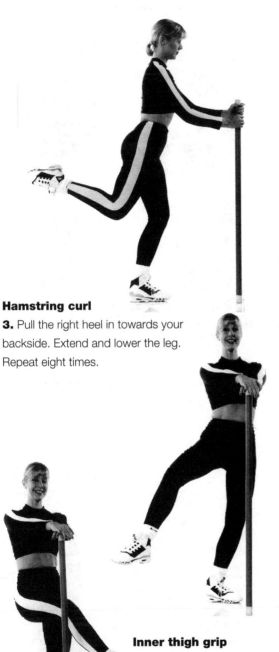

Hamstring curl

3. Pull the right heel in towards your backside. Extend and lower the leg. Repeat eight times.

Inner thigh grip and lift

4. From behind, turn the right leg out to the side, rotating from your hip. Your knee is now towards the ceiling.

Calf Raises

Muscles targeted: *soleus, gastrocnemius, tibalis anterior, foot arch*

Use a chair or broom handle for support and a telephone directory to stand on.
Stand on the directory with your feet close together. Abdominals are contracted and the tailbone is down.

1. Lift on to your toes so that your heels are high off the directory.

2. Lower the heels over the edge of the directory and towards the floor. Lift back up to raised heel. Repeat eight to sixteen times.

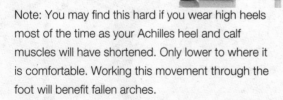

Note: You may find this hard if you wear high heels most of the time as your Achilles heel and calf muscles will have shortened. Only lower to where it is comfortable. Working this movement through the foot will benefit fallen arches.

Inner Thigh Grip

Muscles targeted: *adductors, gluteals*

Stand with your heels together as though you are in a ballet class. Go for a natural turn-out from the hips. Keep your abdominals contracted, chest lifted, the spine lengthened and the tailbone down.
1. Bend your knees slightly.

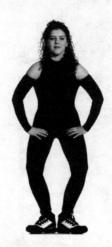
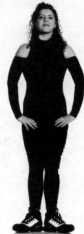

2. Pull up through your inner thighs, gripping them together as you begin to straighten. Press your weight into your heels as you lift.

Body Check

Avoid bending the knees too deeply or leaning forward as you bend.

The Total Lunge and Squat Challenge

Muscles targeted: *gluteals, abductors, quadriceps, hamstrings, calves*

As you squat be conscious of keeping your feet in line with the knees and hips. Keep the tailbone down and the spine lengthened. Maintain a natural curve in the lower back.
The abdominals are contracted, the chest is lifted. Maintain this posture throughout the sequence.

Narrow squat

1. Stand with your feet hip-width apart, squat and lift to standing. Grip the inner thighs and glutes as you lengthen upright. Avoid squatting too deeply, and extend your arms on the squat for balance. Repeat eight times.

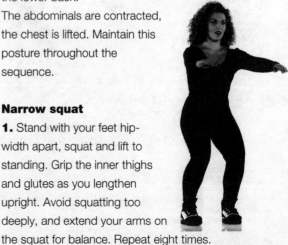

Alternating forward lunges

2. From a narrow squat transfer your weight forward, lifting the leg forward into a lunge. Check your stride length then push off through the ball of your foot back to the narrow squat. Repeat the lunge with the other leg. Alternate legs eight times, taking the last lunge into a wide squat.

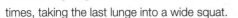

Wide squat

3. Do eight wide squats, maintaining a good posture. Avoid squatting too low, then progress into a squat and lift.

Squat and lift

4. Taking your left leg out to the side, squat and lift eight times with the left leg. Keep your abdominals contracted, and avoid lifting the leg too high.

Backward lunges

5. Return to a narrow squat, hands on the hips and lunge backwards. Alternate the legs. Repeat eight times.

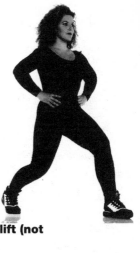

Body check

Avoid striding back too far or bending the knee too deeply. Maintain your exercise posture.

Wide stance, squat and lift (not illustrated)

6. Repeat the wide squats and side leg lifts with the right leg eight times (see stages 3 and 4).

◀ Heel raises

7. Using the narrow squat stance with the feet close together, add heel raises. Squat slightly, then rise, pulling your arms into your sides. Grip your inner thighs as you lift. Repeat eight times.

Forward extension and lift ▶

8. From the narrow squat stance extend your right leg up and forward. Extend your arms for balance. Keep your leg below hip level, return to a small squat then extend the left leg forward. Repeat eight times on alternate legs.

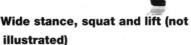

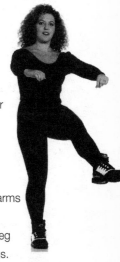

Beginners: follow this routine in two stages. One day do stages 1 and 2, the next try stage 3 on both legs!

Advanced: when this is too easy, do not go for too many sets, instead add resistance by using a body bar or Exer Tube for maximum overload.

Body check

Avoid lifting the leg too high or leaning backwards. This is a very long sequence and it is important to maintain your exercise posture throughout. Focus on the muscle action, gripping the inner thighs and squeezing the glutes as you lift out of a squat. Avoid any discomfort in the knees.

Lying Leg Combo

Muscles targeted: *predominately the abductor*

Preparation

Lie on your side, resting your head on your underarm, abdominals pulled in. The other arm supports the body from rolling forward. The lower leg is bent slightly forward, the top leg is extended outwards in line with your hip and shoulder. The hips are aligned with each other (or stacked), do not let the top hip roll forward. The tailbone is in line with the spine, not jutting backwards.

Low Leg Lift

1. Lift the leg 6–9ins off the floor, keeping the leg level with the hip bone. As you lift, focus on keeping the leg at this level. Press the leg upwards, then squeeze the inner thighs together. Lift on count one, lower on count two. Repeat sixteen times.

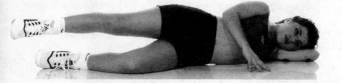

Body check

This is a very controlled movement, so work smoothly and slowly.

2. Progress from above by extending the top leg forward in line with the bent knee. Lift and lower the leg, but not too high. You are lifting on a diagonal from the hip. Feel the outer thigh do the work. The movement should be smooth and controlled. Repeat eight times.

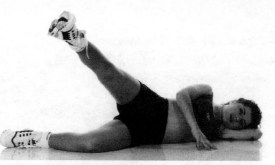

Take two counts to lift and two counts to lower.

3. Hold the leg in a lifted position then bend the knee slightly. Maintain this hold keeping the leg lifted, slightly lift and lower the leg, pulsing up and down 4ins for eight repetitions. Squeeze up on each lift. Finally, lower the leg, extend it out (as in step 1) and repeat the sequence.

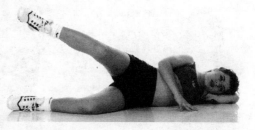

Inner Thigh Lift

Muscle targeted: *adductor*

4. Give the top leg a rest. Let it stretch out over to the floor. Keep your hips stacked on top of each other, do not let them roll. Extend out the lower leg and do inner thigh lifts. Focus on squeezing the thigh upwards. Lift on count one, hold on counts two and three, and lower on count four.

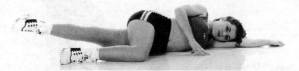

Beginners: eight to sixteen repetitions on each leg.
Advanced: sixteen to twenty-four repetitions, then start the whole sequence again. Repeat twice on each leg. 1kg leg weights or resistance bands can be used.

Rotated Glute and Abductor Squeeze

Muscles targeted: *gluteals, abductors*

(Not for beginners or if you are prone to sciatica).

1. Kneel on all fours on a mat in the box position. Keep your knees apart in line with your hips and your arms extended to the floor, resting on your palms in line with your shoulders. Spread your weight over the supporting leg and arms. Keep your abdominals contracted throughout the exercise. Place your hands directly under the shoulders, knees in line with the hips. Rotate your working leg out sideways from the hip bending the knee, and allowing the heels to touch.

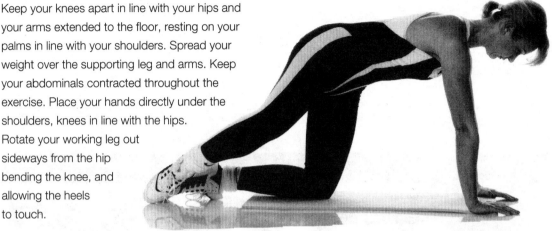

2. Now lift, leading with the outer thigh and knee. Keep your foot slightly lower than the knee and press into your backside. Avoid lifting the knee too high.

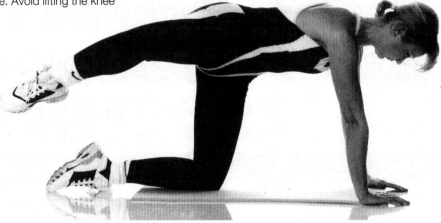

Work up to eight repetitions for each leg.

Body check

Do not rotate the hip. As you move, simply lift and squeeze. Please note this is not a fast or high movement. Do not let the back drop or arch and the abdominals need to be contracted throughout.

Bums

KEEP THEM

▶ FIRM ▶ PERT ▶ SHAPELY ▶ TONED
▶ DON'T SIT AROUND ALL DAY ▶ SQUATS & LUNGES ARE SOME
OF THE BEST TONING EXERCISES YOU CAN DO

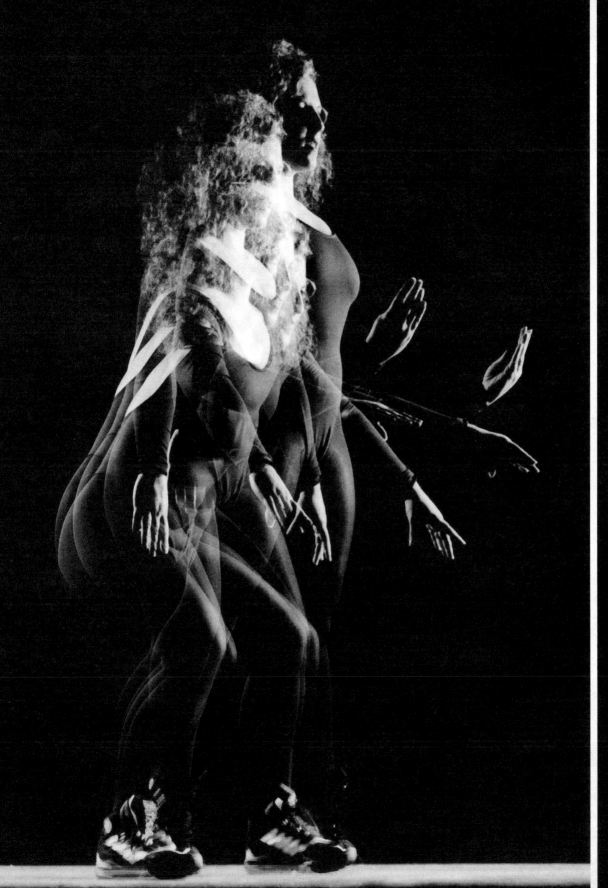

BUM FACTS

Your buttocks, or gluteal muscles, often referred to as the bum, butt, buns or tush, are the most sensual muscle groups on your body. Having a firm backside is one of the biggest turn-ons for men or women.

The size and shape of your buttock muscles is dictated by genes. These determine how prominent the glute muscles are, or how they will develop when exercised.

Through sheer hard work you will achieve a firm, toned bum. Sitting around all day does not help these muscles or cellulite, so keep active whenever possible. Your glute muscles love stair climbing, cycling, jogging, walking and especially hill-walking and aerobics.

The following exercises target the gluteal muscles and in some cases your pelvic floor muscles – the internal muscle group that connects your vaginal, urethra and anal muscles. The pelvic floor muscles should be worked on to enhance your sex life and to prevent prolapse of the womb. These muscles are best worked on their own, while the surrounding gluteal muscles are relaxed, but you can work on them as a bonus during some of these exercises. Look out for the asterisk (*).

Squat and Squeeze

Muscles targeted: gluteals maximus, gluteus medius, hamstring, quadriceps

1. Stand tall with the feet parallel, abdominals contracted, chest lifted, and the spine long. Maintain a natural curve in the lower back.

2. Imagine you are going to sit in a chair. Keep your weight centred over your heels. As you squat, extend your arms out at shoulder level. Exhale on the effort. Focus on contracting the gluteals, inner thighs and quads when returning to standing.

Body check

Avoid squatting too deeply or bending from the waist when you squat.

Beginners: may want to keep hands on the hips. Ten repetitions.

Advanced: aim for two repetitions of sixteen.

Weighted Squat (advanced only)

Using hand weights or a body bar you can increase your muscle work. Hold the weight at your hips, feet are parallel, abdominals are contracted and the tailbone is down.

1. Squat down, focusing on keeping the knees in line over the toes. Press your weight into your heels. As you return to standing, focus on squeezing the glutes together. Repeat sixteen times. The final stage is the extended weighted squat.

Extended Weighted Squat (advanced only)

Extend the bar or weights out to shoulder level. Work up to sixteen repetitions. Avoid any lower back pressure by continually contracting your abdominals. Do not lean backwards or lift the arms too high.

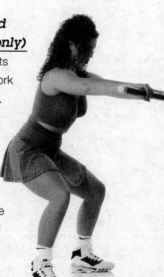

Pelvic Wave *

Muscles targeted: gluteals, abdominals, adductors, pelvic floor

This is a subtle, sensual exercise.

1. Begin by standing with your feet close together and parallel. Turn your feet out slightly from the hips. The abdominals are relaxed to begin with. Allow your tailbone to be in a neutral position so it is not jutting backwards but pointing downwards.

2. Bend your knees then contract your abdominals and roll your pelvis forward and up towards you as you pull up to standing (think of a belly dancer). Squeeze your buttock muscles together as you lift.

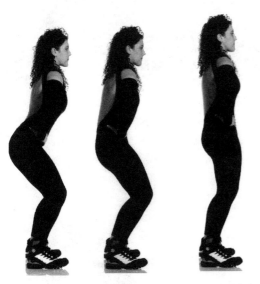

Body check

Keep the action smooth and controlled. It is a very subtle movement but it targets your gluteal and pelvic floor muscles if you focus on pulling them in and upwards as you tilt the pelvis towards you. Work up to sixteen repetitions.

Basic Plié *

Muscles targeted: gluteals, quadriceps, abductors, adductors

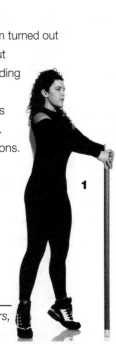

Preparation

Use a chair or pole for support. Stand tall with your feet slightly wider than shoulder-distance apart. The feet are turned out and aligned with your knees. Your tailbone is down to maintain a natural curve in the lower back. The knees are bent, the abdominals pulled in and the chest is lifted.

1. As you bend your knees keep them turned out and only go as low as possible without changing your body alignment or bending your knees past your toes. Focus on contracting your inner thighs, buttocks and pelvic floor muscles as you lift up.
Beginners: work up to twelve repetitions.
Advanced: aim for twenty-four repetitions.

Body check

Avoid any knee or back pain.
Now progress to a plié and rise.

Plié and Rise ▶

Muscles targeted: gluteals, adductors, abductors, gastrocnemius, soleus

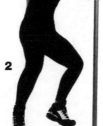

1. As before, but this time from the basic plié, rise up on to your toes, squeezing your inner thighs and glutes together as you lift.

2. Plié into the raised position, bending the knees but keeping the heels off the floor.

3. Then finally lower the heels back down into the plié position.
Beginners: six repetitions.
Advanced: eight to sixteen repetitions.

Body check

Avoid any pressure on the knees. Keep the abdominals contracted all the time and tailbone lengthened down.

Note: Working your gluteal muscles is intense work, shake out between exercises to allow your blood flow to re-energize the muscles.

Rotated Single Leg Glute Squeeze

1. Stand with the legs wide, turning out one leg from the hip. Centre your weight. Lift your heel off the ground. Now do a demi-squat by bending your supporting leg, keeping your heel in line with the toes. Do not bend too deeply. Focus on pressing your weight over your supporting leg.
2. Squat in a slow, controlled way then return to standing. Pull up through your inner thighs and gluteal muscles as you rise.

Body check

Keep your lower spine in a neutral position and the abdominals contracted. Avoid knee discomfort.

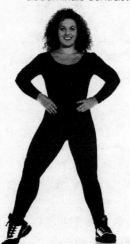
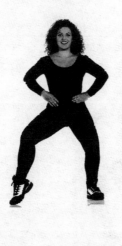

Pelvic Thrust Combo *

Muscles targeted: *gluteals, hamstrings*

Beginners should gradually work their way through this sequence. It looks easy yet the muscle work is intense. It gets really tough at the end.

1. Lie on your back with your knees bent, arms by your side. Contract your abdominals. Allow your pelvis to lift and tilt inwards. Squeeze your inner thighs, glutes and pelvic floor muscles together as you do this, then lower slightly – do not let the lower back or buttocks touch the floor. Repeat the lift and lower sixteen times.

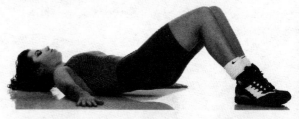

2. As above, but increase the intensity of the exercise by lifting a leg and rotating the knee outwards. Rest the foot just below the supporting knee. Repeat the lift and lower sequence eight times.

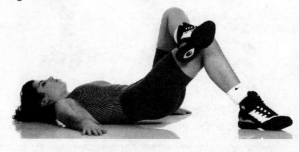

3. Increase the intensity with an extended leg – this is not for beginners. If you start to feel any pressure in the lower back or a burning sensation in the glutes it is time to rest. Squeeze, lift and lower ten times on the same leg then take the extended leg on to stage 4.

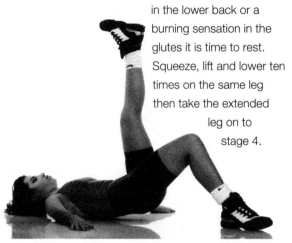

4. Finally, only for the really strong. Bring the legs together, pressing the knees together. Hold this position, lifting and lowering ten times. Keep your abdominals contracted throughout.

Body check

This is tough. You will not be able to lift so high because your glute and hamstring muscles have really overloaded. Release from the exercise if you feel your hamstring cramping. Now repeat the whole sequence from 1–4 on the other leg.

Rotated Glute Squeeze

Muscles targeted: gluteals, tensor fasciae latae

Preparation

This exercise is not suitable if you have had a sciatica problem. Lie sideways with your feet together, the abdominals contracted and your knees together and bent at a slight angle to the hip bone – not 90°. Your head should be resting in line with the spine on the extended under arm, with the other hand placed in front for support.

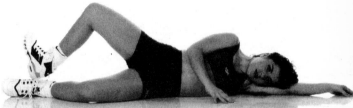

1. Keeping the heels together, rotate the top leg upwards. Feel the muscle tension in the glute, then rotate the knee back down towards the floor.
Beginners: eight repetitions.
Advanced: sixteen repetitions on one leg, carry on to a rotated squeeze.

Body check

There should be no strain in the lower back.

2. Rotate the leg back and hold it there. Allow the heels to separate and,

(cont. over page)

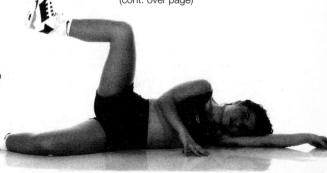

keeping the leg in a fixed position, allow the knee to be pulled in towards your shoulder. The knee is facing up towards the ceiling. Press the heel back to the lower leg, keeping the working leg rotated throughout the movement. Think of squeezing the knee into you then press the heel down. You will feel the tension deep inside the gluteal muscles. Repeat ten times then lower the heels together and rotate the leg forward, back to the resting knee.

3. Sit up and change legs. Repeat the whole sequence twice on each leg.

Lying Butt Squeeze

Muscles targeted: gluteals, hamstring

Preparation

Place a folded towel or thin cushion directly under your pelvis. Lie face down with your head resting on your arms so the neck is lengthened. Squeeze your buttocks together.

1. Curl one leg in, with the foot flexed up to the ceiling. Lift and lower slightly, pulsing the heel towards the ceiling.

Note: This is a very small movement. Feel your glute contract like mad as you lift and squeeze. You can also pull in your pelvic floor muscles from this position. Work up to twenty-five repetitions.

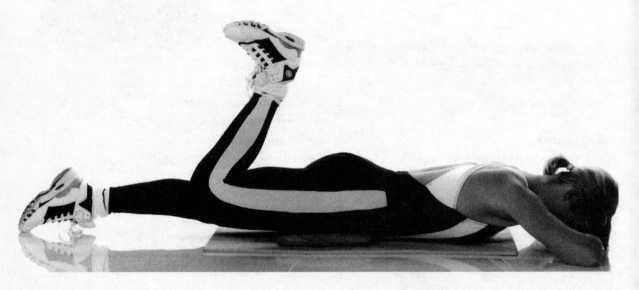

2. This is exactly the same exercise but on all fours. Keep your elbows in line with your shoulder and the abdominals contracted throughout the exercise. Rest the supporting knee on a mat, keep the leg in line with the hip. Take the other leg up, bend at the knee and flex the heel towards the ceiling.

Body check
Avoid any lower-back strain which will happen if you lift the leg too high.

3. Now focus on squeezing and curling the heel inwards (approximately 6ins) towards your buttocks, lift, curl in, release and lower slightly. Repeat sixteen times and change on to the other leg.

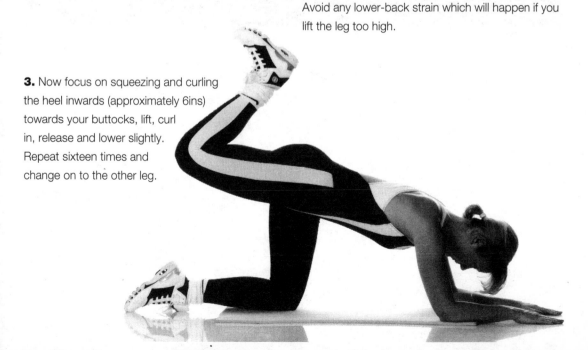

Tums

▶ **FIRM** ▶ **TAUT**

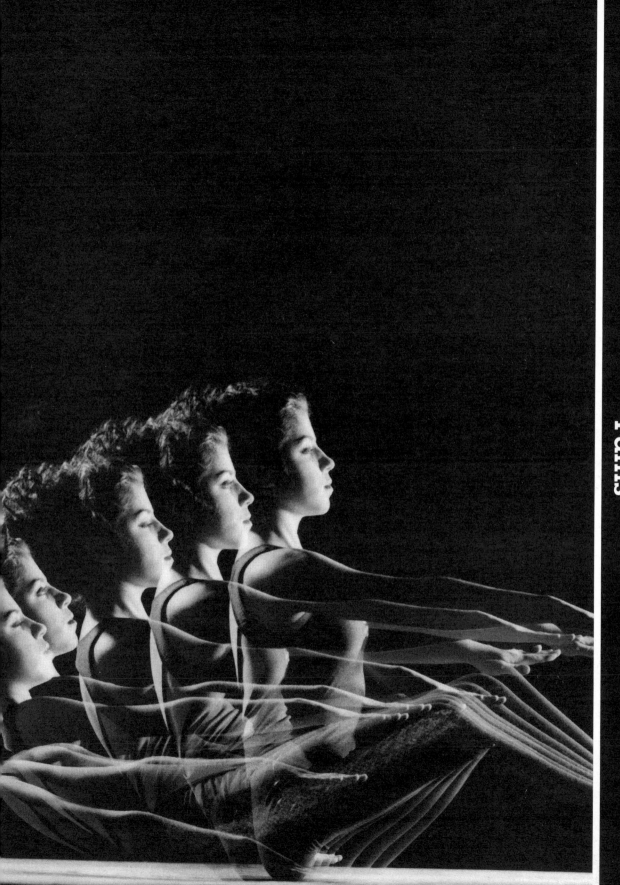

Tums

TUM FACTS

- A completely flat stomach is a myth.
- The abdominal muscles consist of four major muscle groups – the rectus abdominus, external obliques, internal obliques and the transverse abdominus.
- It is natural to deposit fat in the tum area. Even the thinnest of women have a slight tum.
- The washboard stomach look you see on a fit man is rarely achieved in women. It is predominately obtained by unnaturally low body fat, excessive training and genetics.
- Our tum size changes through age and is affected by hormonal changes during our monthly cycle.
- Weak abdominal muscles lead to postural problems and back pain.
- Most of us are only aware of our abdominal muscles when we lie down on the floor to do an abdominal work-out. When we are standing, walking and sitting we rarely focus on pulling in our abdominals.

Before you begin the tum work-outs you need to know exactly where your abdominal muscles are, and how they hold and support your torso when you are standing, sitting and lying down.

Standing

Stand with your feet hip-width apart. Let your tum go completely, you may feel pressure or tension in the lower back.

Now, with your knees slightly bent, place your hands on your hip bones and gently rock your pelvis, tilting inwards and backwards. Focus on lengthening your tailbone so that it points downwards. You'll find your pelvis settles in a neutral position with a slight curve to the spine. The pelvis is not tipped forward or backward, it is central, or in the middle. Avoid clenching your buttocks. Take a deep breath and allow your tum to expand outwards, do not move your pelvic position. Now exhale and contract your tum inwards using your abdominal muscles, pulling in towards the spine. Whenever you are standing, practise finding the upright neutral position. Be conscious of contracting those abs to keep your pelvis in place when walking, talking, carrying or waiting in a queue.

Sitting

Let it all hang out. Notice how your upper body slumps downwards. Now contract your abdominals and lengthen the spine. Lift your ribs out of your pelvis.

It is your abdominal muscles that are lifting your upper body weight and supporting the spine.

Lying

You need to be able to find that neutral position again.

Roll onto your back. Lie there with your knees bent, feet hip-width apart. Look straight up at the ceiling. In this position you may find that your lower back is slightly arched off the ground. This depends how large a curvature of the lower back you have. You will notice this even more when your legs are lying flat on the floor.

Focus on your pelvis. Move it towards you, tilting it inwards so that the lower back is pressed into the floor. This was the position teachers used to instruct you to maintain throughout an abdominal section, with your back continually pressed into the floor. Research has now shown that excessive flattening of the lower back is not natural or good for the lower vertebra discs, so find your neutral lying position.

Now rotate your pelvis away from you to an extreme. This feels awkward and uncomfortable for the lower back. To find the midline, or neutral position, ease your pelvis back and forth, tilting inwards and outwards, keeping your buttocks relaxed as you do this.

Now focus on the midway point where you feel

comfortable. It is a very subtle feeling and because of this it will take time to develop awareness of the neutral position.

If you have extremely tight hamstrings you may find it hard to tilt the pelvis inwards. Do not give up, simply bring your feet in closer to your body throughout the exercises, or even keep your feet placed on a low step or box 4–6ins/10–15cms high as you work-out.

> Tight hamstrings need daily stretching of the hip flexors. Do the Quad and Hip Release on page 118. This condition often arises from too much desk work.

Breathing

When you breathe in, your abdominals will expand like a balloon. As you breathe out, your abdominals are sucked in as you contract inwards and upwards. Focus on breathing out during the hardest part of each exercise, on the lift. When you lift your abdominals are contracting, inwards and upwards. This may sound complicated but in time it will become natural.

Hand placement

Your hands should support the head as you lift, and should not be clamped behind the head crunching the neck which causes pressure on the cervical spine. Place your thumbs behind each ear with your fingers spread wide to cradle the head.

If you have always found that your neck aches after a while doing abdominal work, this is due to the fact that you have led with your head when you curl, and not from the pelvis. After so many repetitions the neck will feel strained. You may have worked with your hands behind your head, pulling your chin into your chest as you curled, creating excessive strain on the neck. You need to be aware of keeping a gap between your chin and chest. Aim for a fist distance apart.

There is a lot to think about but get it right and you will get results!

Warning:

There is a notion that doing hundreds of abdominal crunches a day will give you the flat stomach you have always dreamt of. You can do as many as you like but crunches will not remove spare tyres of fat, loose or saggy skin. A certain proportion of excess fat will disappear with aerobic exercise. For the majority of you mums out there, there is no solution to losing all that post-pregnancy excess skin unless you go under the surgeon's knife. Personally, I am happy with my motherhood tum after four enormous, beautiful, healthy babies!

When you are doing abdominal crunches, focus on starting the curl from your abdominals, contracting them in and allowing the pelvis to tilt inwards, moving the lower back from a neutral position into the floor. Keep your shoulders wide.

This action will happen naturally as long as you focus on curling your body upwards from the pelvis. Most people have a tendency to pull up from their neck, leading with their head and hunching their shoulders.

Wrong

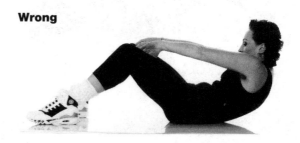

Right

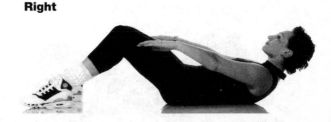

Abdominal Warm Up

Muscles targeted: *abdominals*

Roll-ins

1. Begin in an upright position with your hands placed under your knees.

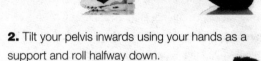

2. Tilt your pelvis inwards using your hands as a support and roll halfway down.

3. Roll back up. Exhale on the roll down. Keep your action smooth. Repeat four times.

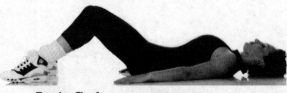

4. Then roll right down.

5. Allow your pelvis to move into neutral.

Basic Curl

Muscle targeted: *rectus abdominus*

1. Place your hands for support at the side of your head, thumbs under the ear and fingers spread wide. Curl up, pulling in your abdominals as the pelvis tilts inwards. Exhale on the effort.

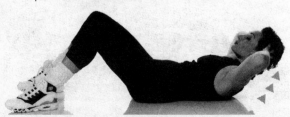

Beginners: twelve repetitions.

Advanced: twenty-four repetitions.

Body check

Avoid crunching the neck. Only curl up until you feel your shoulder blades peeling off the floor.

Reverse Curl Warm Up

Muscles targeted: *rectus abdominus, iliopsoas*

1. Lying on your back, bring your knees up. Turn out the left leg and rest the foot on the right leg. Use your left hand as a support.

2. Contracting your abdominals, roll your pelvis inwards and slowly release.

Body check

Avoid arching the lower back or swinging the legs on the release.

3. Exhale on the effort and pull in your abdominal muscles. Add more resistance with your left hand once you are used to the action.

Beginners: eight repetitions.

Advanced: twelve repetitions then change legs. Aim to do two to three sets.

5. Stretch out allowing the spine to release.

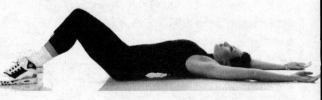

Leg Extensions with Pelvic Tilt

Muscle targeted: *rectus abdominus*

For this exercise you will need a broom handle or weighted pole such as a Body Bar.

1. Begin lying on your back with the pole across your pelvis.

2. Contracting your abdominals, extend one leg down along the floor.

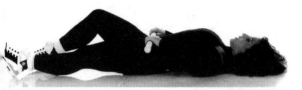

3. Continue to contract harder, allowing your pelvis to tilt inwards as your leg lifts off the floor a few inches. Hold for four counts, exhale on the effort, then lower. Repeat with the other leg.

Beginners: aim for three to four repetitions each leg.

Advanced: up to eight repetitions each leg.

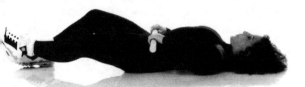

Curl Up 'n' Pulse

Muscle targeted: *rectus abdominus*

For the advanced – a toughie!

1. Beginning in a neutral position, contract the abdominals, and tilt the pelvis forwards. Using your hands, crawl up your thighs, peeling your shoulders off the floor into a comfortable curl. The hands are helping to support your upper-body weight.

Allow the elbows to bend and curl in, bringing your ribs into your pelvis.

Focus on pulling

your pubic bone in towards your naval.

2. Ouch! It is hard now as it is static work! Contract even more and let go of your thighs, allow your feet to flex and reach to your knees. Lifting and lowering slightly, curl and pulse eight times, working up to sixteen. Advanced can go for more. To pulse means small contractions where you continually curl inwards, release slightly and then curl again.

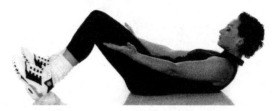

Body check

Avoid any neck crunching or shoulder hunching.

Basic Reverse Curl

Muscle targeted: *rectus abdominus*

1. Lie on your back with your feet together, knees bent and your legs lifted towards the ceiling. Contract your abdominal muscles to pull in and slightly lift your lower half. Exhale then release. Beginners place your palms face down by the side of your hips for support.

Beginners: at least eight repetitions.

Advanced: two sets of sixteen.

Body check

Avoid swinging the legs.

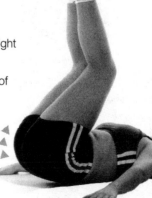

Extended Curl

Muscle targeted: *rectus abdominus*

1. Position yourself as in basic curl. The knees are bent, the pelvis is in neutral, support your head with one hand and leave the other arm extended behind you.

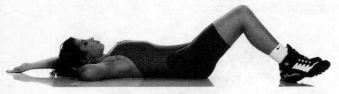

2. Contract your abdominals. Curl up, allowing the pelvis to tilt inwards and leaving your arm behind you on the lift.

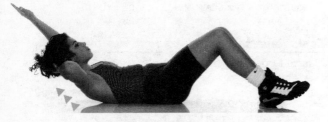

3. Then hold and extend the arm to your knee.

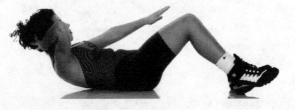

Keep contracting throughout this time. Bring your arm back behind your ear, then lower the torso. Exhale on the various efforts. It is a slow smooth action.

Beginners: eight repetitions changing arms after four.

Advanced: eight repetitions with each arm. Aim to do two sets.

Reverse Curl and Squeeze

Muscle targeted: *rectus abdominus*

1. In this version, you are gripping a cushion with your legs. The focus on the curl is now deeper. Curl in as before.

> **Beginners:** up to twelve repetitions.
> > **Advanced:** aim to do three sets of twelve. This exercise is great for mothers.

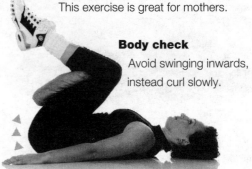

Body check
Avoid swinging inwards, instead curl slowly.

Frog Curl and Reach

1. This is another exercise where the hip flexors are put out of action. Allow your knees to open to the sides. You may find your back arching in this position if you are not very flexible. If this is the case, place your feet apart and flat on the floor with your knees facing the ceiling.

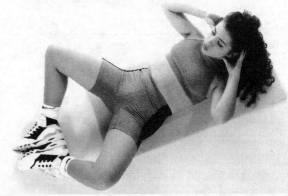

Support your head in your hands. Contract your abdominals then curl up and reach through your legs. Bring your hands back to your head for the roll down.

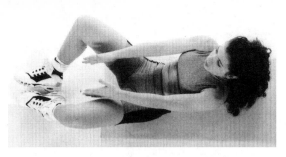

Beginners: work up to eight to sixteen repetitions, remembering to exhale on the effort.
Advanced: go for two sets.

Reverse Curl and Squeeze Combo

Muscle targeted: rectus abdominus

1. This time place your hands along the floor above your head, gripping the cushion with your legs. Reverse curl ten times. Beginners will need to keep their hands by their hips. Stay at level 1 repeat ten times. Work up to two sets.

2. Taking the hands to the side of the head for support, reverse curl and hold in. Now add an upper body curl by curling up from your shoulders, holding your elbows out wide.

3. Progress to a double crunch, contracting even more, and taking your elbows towards your knees. A double crunch is where you pull in your lower and upper body together. Avoid pulling the neck, feel the muscle work increase.

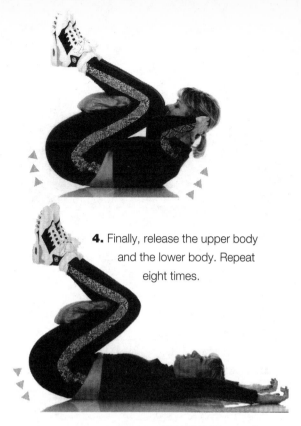

4. Finally, release the upper body and the lower body. Repeat eight times.

Weighted waist shaper

Muscles targeted: obliques, rectus abdominus

Beginners: do not use the weights and keep one hand on the floor for support.

1. Lying flat on your back, hold a 2–3kg weight by the right shoulder with the left hand. The right hand is cradling the head for support. Contract the abdominals.

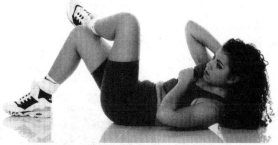

2. Curl across, rotating the body to the opposite shoulder and towards the opposite knee. Exhale.

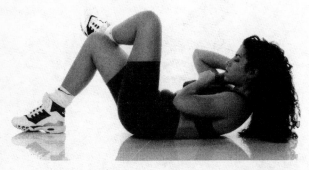

3. Rotate to the centre, keep your abdominals contracted then rotate across again towards the opposite knee.

Beginners: repeat eight times before releasing. Repeat on other side.

Advanced: repeat sixteen to twenty-four times. Repeat on other side.

Body check

Avoid crunching the neck by keeping the abdominals contracted throughout the repetitions.

Extended Oblique

Muscles targeted: *internal and external obliques*

1. Curl up and rotate as in Waist Shaper (page 111) but this time take both your hands to the opposite shoulder across towards the knee.

Beginners: you may need to support your head with one arm. Simply curl up, rotate, reach, then curl down. Do six repetitions on alternate sides.

Advanced: Lift and lower slightly, pulsing eight to twelve times. Do three sets on alternate sides.

Body check Avoid neck strain.

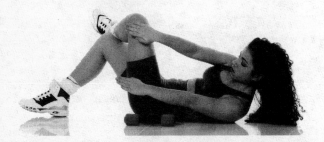

Chair Combo

Muscle targeted: *rectus abdominus*

Using a chair isolates the abdominal muscles so you work harder and deeper.

1. Spread your fingers either side of your head. Contract your abdominals, allowing the pelvis to tilt inwards then curl up. Exhale on the lift, avoiding neck crunching.

Beginners: aim for three sets of eight repetitions.

Advanced: aim to do three sets of fifteen repetitions.

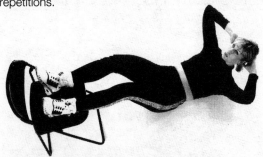

Curl and Rotate

Muscles targeted: *rectus abdominus, obliques*

This exercise is suitable for beginners because the head is supported.

1. With the fingers supporting the head, curl up and take one opposite shoulder towards the opposite knee. Exhale, return to the centre and roll down.

Beginners: sixteen repetitions.

Advanced: two sets of sixteen repetitions on alternate sides.

Body check

Is your lower back still in contact with the floor when you curl? Avoid any neck pulling.

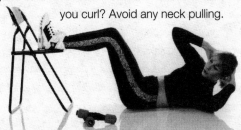

Rope Climb

Muscle targeted: *rectus abdominus*

Not suitable for beginners.

1. From the basic curl extend your arms up in front of you. Imagine you are climbing a rope. Reach up and pull your body up slightly as you reach with alternating arms.

Beginners: repeat sixteen times then curl back and release.

Advanced: repeat sixteen to twenty-four times then curl back and release.

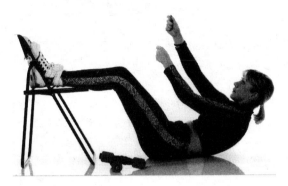

Body check

Is there a gap between the chin and chest? Are you focusing on contracting the abdominals and pressing them into the floor?

Weighted Curl

Muscle targeted: *rectus abdominus*

Not suitable for beginners.

Finally, overload those rectus abdominal muscles with a weighted curl. Use a handweight or a plastic bottle filled with water for added resistance.

1. Begin as for the basic curl but hold the weight above your head on the floor.

2. Focus on contracting your abdominals, allowing the pelvis to tilt in as you curl up, leaving your arms above you and the weight just above the head. Exhale on the effort.

Beginners: aim to do twelve times.

Advanced: repeat sixteen times and work up to two sets.

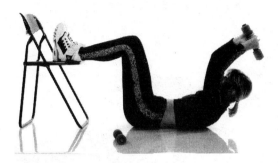

Body check

Keep the action smooth and controlled. Beginners: once you are familiar with the chair combo, move on to the advanced exercises and repeat the whole sequence two to three times.

Reverse Chair Strengthener

Muscle targeted: *rectus abdominus*

Not for beginners.

This exercise looks so simple but it requires a great deal of strength. It targets the lower abdominal area to the maximum with a static contraction.

1. Begin with your feet resting on a chair, with the shoulders and back relaxed.

2. Focus on contracting your abdominals into the floor, allowing the pelvis to rotate inwards. Pull in so much you lift your heels 2–4ins off the chair. Exhale on the effort and hold for a minimum of ten seconds, longer if possible. Then lower one heel at a time, repeat four to eight times.

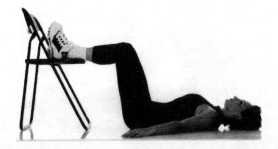

Body check

Keep your hip angle at 90° for maximum effort. If you feel your lower back arching stop the exercise, as you are not yet strong enough.

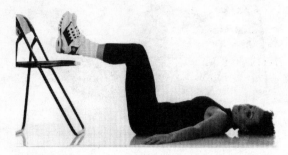

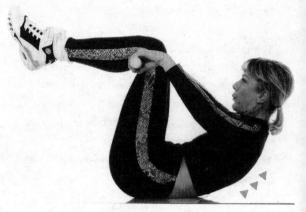

Bar Curl Ups

Muscle targeted: rectus abdominus

Not suitable for beginners.
For this exercise you will need a Body Bar or broom handle.

1. Lying on your back, place the bar behind your knees and hold on to the bar at either side of your knees.

2. Focusing on contracting the abdominals, turn your elbows outwards as you curl up. Do sixteen repetitions.

Weighted Reverse Curl

Muscle targeted: rectus abdominus

Not suitable for beginners.
Hold the bar in place by gripping it behind the knees. Contract your abdominals as you curl inwards, allowing your butt to lift a couple of inches off the floor. Aim to do eight to sixteen repetitions.

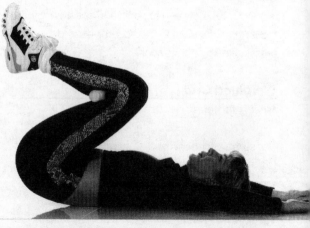

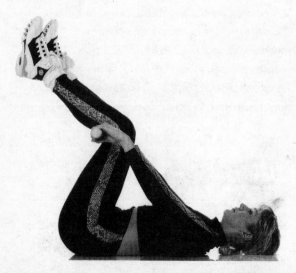

Body check

Avoid lifting the shoulders as you curl the lower body.

Weighted Curl Up

Muscle targeted: *rectus abdominus*

Not suitable for beginners.
You can use a light hand weight for this exercise.
Lie as for bar curl, but with the bar above your head.
Focus on contracting your abdominals then curl the
bar up over your head towards your knees. Aim to
do two sets of sixteen repetitions.

Body check

Do not use momentum to lift to the bar. Lift it in a
controlled way as you curl.

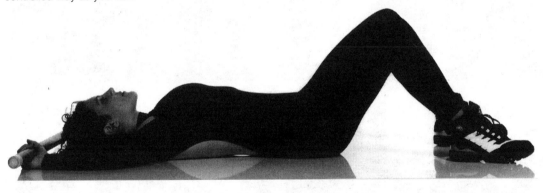

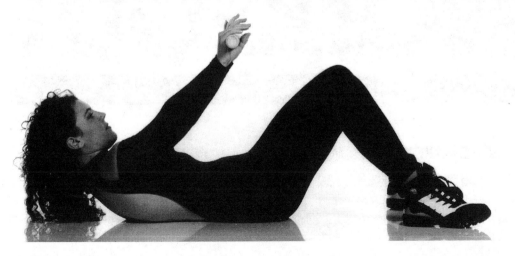

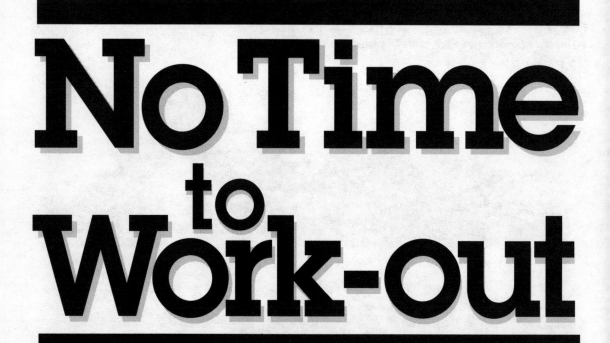

No Time to Work-out

▶ **FOLLOW THE ULBT TEN MINUTE PLAN** ▶ **DO IT WHILE WATCHING TV**

▶ **DO IT THE MOMENT YOU GET UP** ▶ **NO EXCUSES – JUST DO IT**

No Time to Work-out

he pressure is on. There is no time to do a long work-out but it is still a priority for you. Stop making excuses and simply do it. If you have time to watch TV you have time to work-out, even if it is on the couch – a great place for an abdominal work-out.

Commit yourself by taking the following steps:

▶ Make time. Start with ten-minute blocks once a day. Work up to twice a day. Build up your time block so that eventually you work-out for thirty minutes once a day.

▶ Be creative about where you exercise (try in bed).

▶ While the supper cooks, work-out.

▶ Kids are in the bath – work-out in the hall, leaving the door open so that you can keep a safe eye on them.

▶ Insist you have a fast walk, cycle, run or skate with your partner twenty minutes before dinner. You will both benefit from the feel-good factor afterwards.

▶ Get up earlier by going to bed earlier. Work-out before the day starts.

▶ Keep a tracksuit at work. Try twenty minutes power-walking, or running at lunch time, then grab a sandwich and eat it slowly while you get changed for work again.

▶ Wear a T-shirt and leggings around the house so that when you have a spare moment you can get down to the ten-minute plan.

▶ Make an appointment with yourself. Keep an alarm clock on your desk or wear a watch with an alarm. Set the alarm to tell you it is time to stop working, leave the office and start your exercise. Do not break your appointment with yourself.

▶ Never let forty-eight hours slip by without exercise.

▶ Enjoy the exercise and use the time to focus on your body. If your mind wanders let it focus on your breathing, exercising can be meditative.

▶ Warm up for the ten-minute work-out by either having a short brisk walk, dancing around to your favourite music or jogging around the block for five minutes or so.

THE TEN-MINUTE WORK-OUT

Outer thigh press and lift
Muscles targeted: *adductors, abductors*

1. Lie on your side and bend your lower leg for a stable base. Keep your hips in line with your shoulders and your abdominals contracted inwards throughout the exercise to keep the spine and pelvis stabilized.

2. Begin with the extended top leg. With the knee facing forwards lift the leg to a comfortable height. Avoid bending the lower back or rolling the hips.

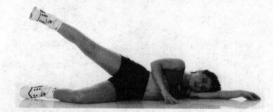

3. As you lower the leg, focus on pressing the leg downwards, squeezing the butt muscles and the inner thighs together. Do not quite touch the floor. As you lift think of pressing the leg away. Feel the muscles do the work.

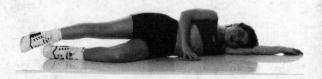

Beginners: sixteen repetitions per leg.
Advanced: work up to twenty-four repetitions per leg. Do two sets.

Body check

Keep the action smooth and controlled.

Waist Shaper

Muscles targeted: rectus abdominus, obliques

1. Lying with your knees bent and arms by your side, curl up, tilting the pelvis inwards. Then reach down one side of your thigh, pulling your ribs towards your hip bone. Return to the centre curl, and reach down the other side. Exhale each time you curl. This exercise looks simple but it is tough.

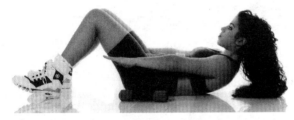

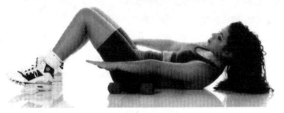

Beginners: may need to support the head on the one hand. Aim to do six each side.
Advanced: work up to ten each side.

Body check

Avoid any neck strain.

Bum & Tum Toner

Muscles targeted: gluteus maximus, adductors, rectus abdominas

1. Place a cushion between your legs, and hold it in place by squeezing your inner thighs. Contract your abdominals. Tilt the pelvis inwards and squeeze your glute muscles together as you lift. Grip, lift and squeeze.

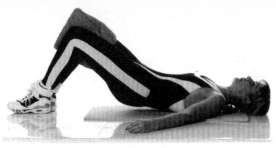

Beginners: fifteen repetitions.
Advanced: work up to twenty-five repetitions.

Body check

Do not lift the backside high.

2. From the butt squeezes, lower the pelvis and go straight into basic curls. Keep squeezing your inner thighs together as you curl up. Repeat the curl sixteen times.

Beginners: repeat the curl sixteen times.
Advanced: work up to twenty-two repetitions.

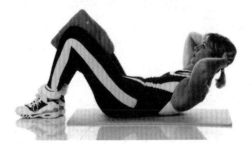

3. Repeat the whole sequence three times.

Body check

Avoid neck crunching; focus on pressing the lower back into the floor as you curl up, exhale on the effort.

Front of Leg Shaper - Quad Lift

Muscles targeted: quadriceps, iliopsoas

Preparation

Lie on your back, then come up so that you are resting on

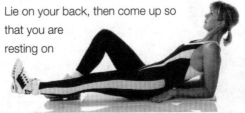

your elbows. Tuck your fingers underneath your lower back and keep the chest lifted.

1. The abdominals are contracted inwards to stabilize the pelvis throughout the exercise. Extending the leg, lift it up to knee line only, then lower.

Beginners: lift and lower eight times.

Advanced: lift and lower sixteen times. 1kg weights can be used.

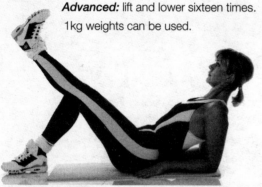

Body check

Be aware that you do not cramp the quad muscles. Slowly lift the leg up then lower, breathing out on the effort. Check that your back does not arch. If your abdominals release, your pelvis will rotate outwards. Avoid straining the neck by sinking down and hunching the shoulders.

Inner Thigh and Abs

Muscles targeted: adductors, abductors, rectus abdominus

1. Start by working on your inner thighs with your legs up in the air, knees slightly bent. The abdominals are contracted to stabilize the back. Open your legs out at a comfortable width, just past your hips. Focus on squeezing in and gripping your buttock muscles as you bring your legs together.

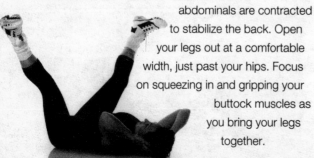

2. Do eight inner thigh squeezes then add eight basic curls as you work the legs. Curl up when the legs are together. Keep your abdominals contracted throughout the exercise.

Beginners: one set.

Advanced: work up to three sets. 1kg leg weights can be used.

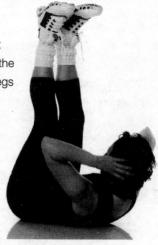

Leg shaper

Muscles targeted: hamstring, calves, gluteals, abdominals

Preparation

On all fours begin by bending the elbows, keeping the knees in line with the hips. Elbows are under your shoulders and abdominals contracted to hold the back in place.

1. Bend one knee towards your chest, then lift it

▲ upwards keeping your foot flexed.

▲ Squeeze into your glute muscles.

▲ There should be no pressure in the lower back. Keep the abdominals contracted throughout this exercise. Avoid lifting the leg too high.

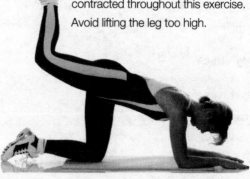

2. Hold the leg up by doing small lifts and squeezes. Pulse eight times.

3. Then extend the leg and lower it back down to the floor.

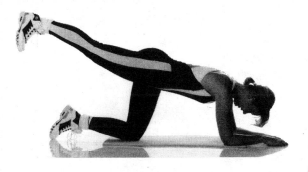

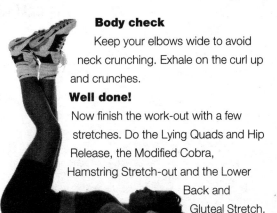

2. Do a reverse curl, contracting your abdominals and allowing the pelvis to tilt inwards, lifting the legs inwards and up. Hold this contraction. Exhale on the contraction.

Beginners: Six repetitions on each leg.
Advanced: Ten repetitions on each leg.
You may want to ease out before you repeat on the other leg.

Body check

Do not lift the leg too high. Avoid bending the lower back and swinging the leg during the lift. Keep the action as a smooth controlled movement. Keep the abdominals contracted throughout the exercise.

3. Now add the upper body curl up and by doing small lifts and squeezes, pulse four times. Focus on bringing your ribs to your pubic bone. Lower the upper body first.

Double Crunch Combo

Muscles targeted: *rectus, abdominus*

1. Begin with your legs up in the air, feet crossed and knees slightly bent. Your head is resting in your hands, the elbows are held slightly wide.

4. Once the upper body is lowered, release the lower body. Repeat the sequence.
Beginners: four repetitions.
Advanced: eight repetitions.

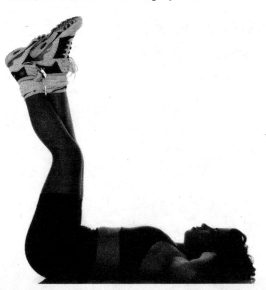

Body check

Keep your elbows wide to avoid neck crunching. Exhale on the curl up and crunches.

Well done!

Now finish the work-out with a few stretches. Do the Lying Quads and Hip Release, the Modified Cobra, Hamstring Stretch-out and the Lower Back and Gluteal Stretch.

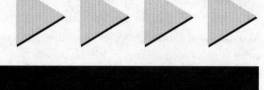

Stretch

▶ **LENGTHEN** ▶ **EASE** ▶ **RELAX**
▶ **RELEASE TENSION**

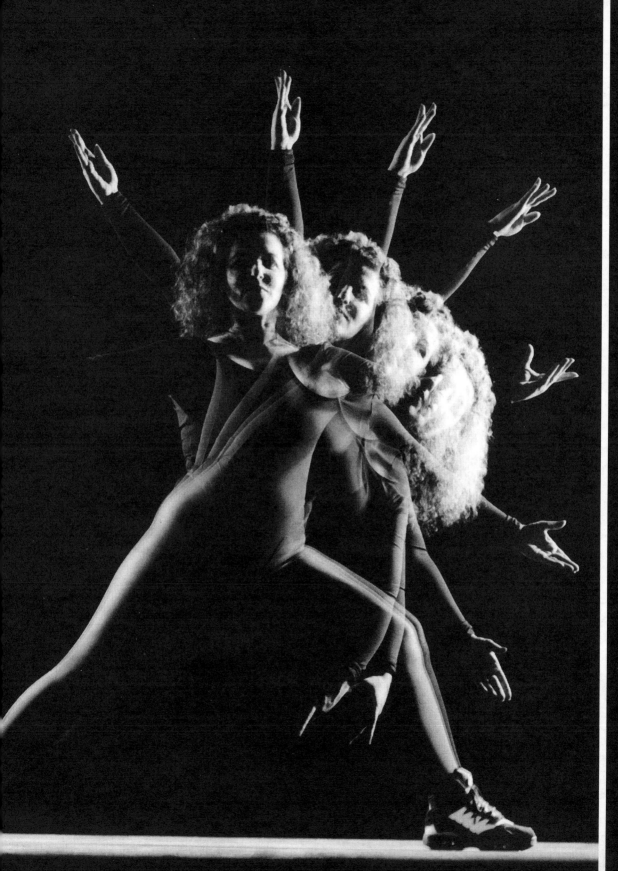

Stretch

Stretch and release

Well done. Now you've completed the programme it is time to stretch and release.

Many people ignore this section in a work-out because it is static and peaceful. It seems like a waste of time but it is vital. No fitness programme can be complete without adding flexibility training or stretching to unite one's mind and body. Dancers and gymnasts are flexible beyond the normal range of movements. Trying to push your body to these extremes is not sensible or realisitic and can lead to serious injury.

Stretching enhances muscle relaxation. The aim of stretching is to increase joint mobility while maintaining joint stability, through static held positions. Stretching relaxes muscles and increases the blood flow to tense muscles. Tensed muscles are contracted, restricting circulation and cutting off vital nutrients and oxygen to muscle cells. This leads to muscle fatigue and pain. Fatigued muscles are unable to absorb the impact, shock and stress of movement. This is when injury can occur.

The muscle soreness that occurs after too intense or too much exercise, can be reduced by stretching or cooling down after intense exercise such as aerobics. Stretching allows peace of mind, offering quiet moments within oneself. It allows time to be in touch with one's feelings and to focus on relaxaing the body and the mind. Stretching improves posture and balances muscle symmetry, allowing greater range of movement of the muscle and joint.

When not to stretch

▶ Before exercising when you are not warm.
▶ Avoid stretching when you are recovering from a severe injury, recently strained ligaments or a sprained muscle.
  Pain in the joint or muscle while stretching is a warning that something is wrong. There may be soft tissue damaged from an injury or infection.
▶ If you suffer from osteoporosis, arthritis, rheumatic disorder or back problems, seek advice from your doctor or a physiotherapist before following a stretching programme.

Pregnant and new mothers

You can easily overstretch during pregnancy because your stretching abilities dramatically increase. This is due to the hormone released that relaxes and softens connective tissue allowing changes in the pelvic movement for birth. Being hyper-flexible while pregnant through yoga stretching does not make the birth any easier. It can cause tremendous stability problems after the birth.

Age and flexibility

Connective tissue shortens as we age. This is natural because of tighter muscles. We start to stiffen up and older people become prone to muscle strain from sudden movement or a forceful jolt. Muscles need to be stretched to minimize the effect of muscle shortening. Regular, gentle stretching is necessary.

How to stretch

1. You need to be warm before stretching. You cannot stretch cold muscles, this only leads to injury. This is why we stretch after a work-out because the body temperature is raised after exercise due to increased circulation.
2. Concentrate on the area or muscle group when stretching, focus on the muscle lengthening.
3. Balance your stretches, do not just do what you feel like. Stretch the whole body, and all of the muscle groups, such as stretching the hamstring (back of leg) then the quadriceps (front of thigh).
4. Do not force or bounce into the stretch.
5. Hold stretches for fifteen to sixty seconds.
6. Stretch to the full range of movement not to the point of pain. As you hold a stretch you will feel the muscle give, then you can stretch further.
7. Stretch before vigorous activity and after a work-out.
8. Be patient, flexibility takes time.

Breathing

As you stretch, focus on deep breathing. Breathe in and out through your nose, allowing your chest to raise and expand as you inhale and to lower and contract as you exhale. Breathing in this way will actually help release muscle tension. Deep breathing increases the oxygen supply to your muscles and improves the circulation, thereby washing out the chemical waste known as lactic acid which occurs in the muscular tissue after exercise. A long deep stretch will help with the lactic acid wash eliminating muscle soreness, leaving you centred and relaxed. *Follow the stretches given here in sequence.*

1. Meditative release

Begin by lying stretched out on the floor with your shoulders relaxed and your arms extended over your head. Focus on deep breathing for a minute or two, inhaling and exhaling through your nose. Feel your breathing rhythm.

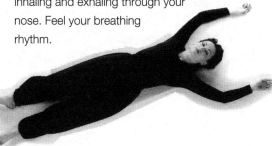

2. Hamstring Stretch-out

a. Bring one knee up to your chest. Place your hands behind the knee to ease the leg in towards you. Breathe deeply.
b. Hold for ten seconds then push your leg away from your body for four seconds, creating a tension by

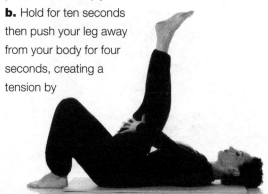

working against your hands. Then stretch the leg in again, easing it closer to your body. Repeat on the other leg.

3. Lower Back and Gluteal Stretch

a. Ease the knee across your body over to the opposite side, using your hand for support if necessary. Allow your lower back and gluteal muscles to release. With one arm pointing back in the opposite direction, turn your neck and head and look along this arm as you stretch. Breathe deeply, avoid stretching too far and hold for fifteen to thirty seconds. When you roll your leg back, help the leg up with the opposite hand.

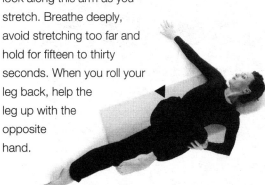

b. Progress the stretch by bending your knees, pointing one leg up towards the ceiling, the other leg rotating outwards from the hip. The knee is bent and the foot is resting on the other leg. Place your arms by your side. This is a gluteal stretch. Ease the legs in towards you until you feel the stretch. Hold for fifteen to twenty seconds.

c. Exhale on the stretch. Repeat the whole sequence on your other leg.

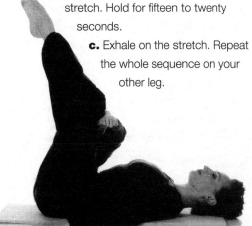

4. Quad and Hip Release

a. Lie on your front with your head turned sideways, shoulders relaxed and your arms pointing forwards.

b. Bend one knee and ease the leg into your buttock. Hold the ankle.

c. Focus into the floor, feel the stretch from the hip flexor and front of the thigh.

Hold the stretch for fifteen to twenty seconds. Avoid pulling from the knee. Repeat on the other leg.

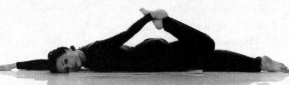

5. Modified Cobra

Take the quad and hip release into a modified cobra. Lengthen the upper body. Raise up on to your hands, resting on your elbows and keeping your chest lifted. Allow your chest to expand as you breathe deeply through your nose. Hold for a count of twenty.

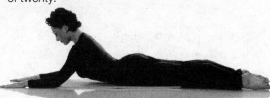

Body check

Avoid lifting too high and causing pressure on your lower back. Check that your neck is an extension of the spine by looking straight ahead and not tipping your head to the side.

6. Prayer Stretch

a. Now ease your body weight backwards by pushing up on your hands into a prayer stretch.

b. To sink down as you round your lower back you need to keep your knees wide apart. Place your arms where they are comfortable. Allow the shoulders to sink as you stretch and continue to breathe through your nose.

Note: because of this position your breathing will appear to be shallower.

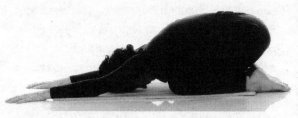

7. Spine Release

a. Take the prayer stretch into a spine release.

b. Resting on your knuckles place your hands approximately 8ins away from your knees. With your hands in line with your shoulders, round up from your shoulder blades in a smooth and controlled movement. Allow the head to follow the spine. As you round your upper back, contract your abdominals in, allowing the pelvis to tilt inwards. Exhale as you do this.

c. In a controlled way slowly release the spine. Flatten the lower back and progress into a natural arch. Avoid dropping the abdominals. Allow your head to follow through the spinal wave. Focus on inhaling in this position. Repeat the exercise four times in a slow, controlled wave.

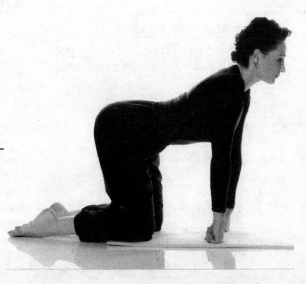

8. The Thinker Abductor Stretch

a. Sit keeping one leg bent and the other extended in front of you. Lifting your chest, reach forward towards the ankle and hold for fifteen to twenty seconds. Focus on deep breathing. Avoid pressing the knee cap of the extended leg downwards.

b. Continue and cross the bent knee over the extended leg, using your hand to support your back as you lift your chest. Ease the bent leg in towards your chest. Feel the stretch in the side of your leg before you rotate your body around. Hold for ten seconds.

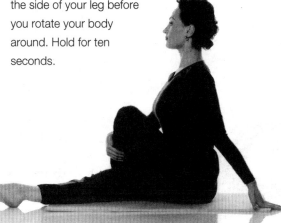

9. Spinal Release

Continue the thinker abductor stretch into a spinal rotation by bringing your supporting hand closer to your back. Let your head follow the spine. Hold and breathe deeply for fifteen seconds. Repeat the sequence on the other leg.

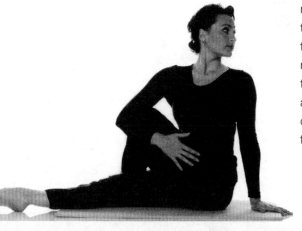

10. Side Stretch

In a seated position, take the legs wide apart, one knee bent and the other leg extended. Point your toes. Ease upwards and over the extended leg with the opposite arm. The other arm supports the weight of your upper body. Keep your abdominals contracted, to hold the back straight and strong. Let your head follow the curve of the spine and keep your chest lifted. Focus on lengthening up and outwards as you breathe deeply. Hold for fifteen to twenty seconds. Repeat on the other side.

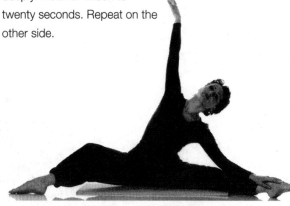

11. Chest Stretch

Sit with your knees bent forward and take your hands behind your hips, resting your weight on your finger tips. Lifting your chest gently ease your shoulders back. Look upwards keeping your mouth closed. Feel the chest open. Hold for eight seconds, then release. Repeat four times then lie flat and breathe deeply on the floor.

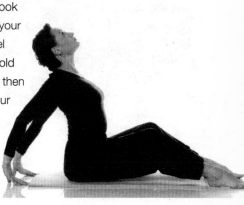

12. Neck Release

a. Sit cross-legged with your weight evenly distributed, your abdominals pulled in and your back straight. Place one hand on the side of your head, supporting your weight and posture by placing one hand by your side. Ease your right ear to your right shoulder. Do not force this as the neck is a stress tension area. Simply breathe deeply and let the tension release. Hold for ten seconds, then slowly return to an upright position. Repeat on the other side.

If you used resistance equipment during the advanced exercises, give your arms a stretch, sitting tall and centred with the abdominals contracted.

13. Deltoid Shoulder Stretch (not illustrated)

Stand straight with the abdominals contracted. Take one arm across the body. This arm is relaxed. Ease it in to your chest with the other hand. Hold for fifteen seconds.

14. Tricep Stretch (not illustrated)

Progress the deltoid shoulder stretch to a tricep stretch for the back of the arms. How far you will be able to bend the arm will depend on your flexibility. Bend the arm over and across the head. Support the arm from either the front as you bend it back behind the head, or hold from behind the head. Hold for fifteen seconds.

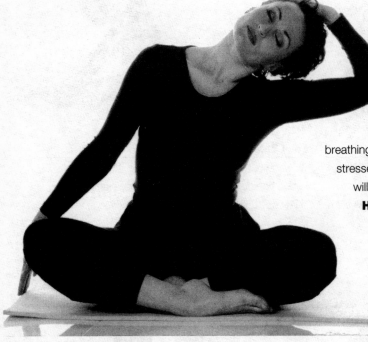

Finally, end your stretch with a relaxation session as you began by lying down on the floor, with all your muscles relaxed and focus on deep breathing for ten minutes.

Let your mind wander and focus on something that makes you really happy. Breathe deeply in and out through your nose feeling your breathing rhythm. Simply drift away from the stresses of life. Ten minutes in a meditative state will enable you to cope with anything. **Happy relaxation.**

Final say

▶ **MAKE FITNESS A PART OF YOUR LIFE FOREVER**
▶ **YOUR SAY** ▶ **CREDIT TO**

FINAL SAY

There you have it, the whole programme. Well done! You now have the resources to make the ULBT programme work for you. If you have come this far I know you are serious. It is so easy to pick up an exercise book, flick through a chapter or two and then forget all your good intentions once life's hectic times take over.

Following an exercise programme from a book is one of the hardest things to do yet it is my only link with you. For all you video fans, the book is designed to complement the ULBT video which is being released.

My message to you is make exercise part of your life, not just a fad or a trend. You may have bought this book to shape up for a special occasion, but do not forget the feel-good factor that comes from having an exercised, firm body. Be active throughout your holidays, weekends and even during your lunch hours. You can be active wherever you are.

Keep your muscles alert by creating your own cross-training. Mix the ULBT programme with other fat-burning activities that you enjoy such as dancing, playing a sport or running.

So where do you go from here? Once you have followed the ULBT programme for several weeks and feel you are fitter and stronger, challenge yourself. Work-out longer, harder, or use resistance equipment to overload your muscles.

The key to maintaining your firm new shape is to always challenge your body. Keep it alert with a mix of exercise and activity. Nourish your body with real foods, adapt your diet to seasonal changes. Enhance your self-esteem with nurturing activities such as the occasional massage. Finally, maintain a healthy body image, learn to love and accept yourself. Always make time for yourself.

Whatever shape or size you are remember: think firm not fat. The energy you gain from the programme will help you live life to the full – whatever happens.

With my final words I've enclosed real life experiences of women from different backgrounds who have changed their attitudes to their lifestyle through the ULBT programme.

Let me know how you get on.

Write to me:
The Editor
Get Active magazine
41 Overstone Road,
Hammersmith,
London W6 0AD
Alternatively, come to one of my events and tell me about it!
Happy exercising.

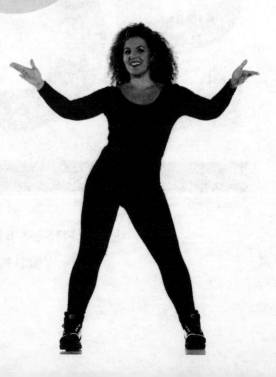

Create your own cross-training diary

	MON	TUE	WED	THUR	FRI	SAT	SUN
Example plan to:	Walking	ULBT	Tennis	ULBT	Dancing, clean house, walk, ULBT	ULBT	Bike ride
ACHIEVED							
Week 1 plan to:								1
ACHIEVED							
Week 2 plan to:								2
ACHIEVED							
Week 3 plan to:								3
ACHIEVED							
Week 4 plan to:								4
ACHIEVED							
Week 5 plan to:								5
ACHIEVED							
Week 6 plan to:								6
ACHIEVED							
Week 7 plan to:								7

YOUR SAY

Kate Ricketts: actress

Lydia's ULBT classes were recommended to me by TV cook Leslie Waters who had been attending her sessions. I went alone, and I was soon hooked, the atmosphere was so unpretentious and there were all shapes, sizes and ages working out together.

Lydia's teaching methods were thorough and she was clear that the programme was tough stuff, yet her fun, entertaining and friendly manner motivated me. Over time I saw my body change. Mentally the exercises enabled me to focus and concentrate better and to build up my stamina. Physically my body became more streamlined.

Now I am better in shape than I had been in my twenties. My advice is to stick to it. Results take time and building up your stamina is important. Only exercise when you feel like it, do not feel guilty if you miss a session. After a while you will actually want to exercise.

Suki Miles: instructor and dancer

I came to Lydia's studio out of curiosity as a teacher hoping to find work. To get noticed I tried out her ULBT class. My whole attitude to exercise changed. For the first time I was focused on body control, alignment and muscular work. I was so used to being in instructor's classes where they simply demonstrated. She's great to watch, she applied all the RSA teaching principles yet taught such in-depth combinations of exercises, allowing one to feel the muscle work before moving on to another sequence. I felt awakened, and in control of what I was doing.

I wanted to learn Lydia's teaching methods, her exercises and more. Luckily I was taken on to teach at her studio. During this time I opened up to her and spoke about my eating problems. I was a professional dancer touring with major bands. When I am busy I am in control, when I am not I would simply binge on everything. I have seen experts for help but I have not been able to come to terms with all my problems. Lydia's ULBT programme has redirected me, I am finding ways of coping with my low self-esteem and body image. Being honest with myself has enabled me to take responsibility for my actions and I am now making more balanced, healthier food choices.

Being a member of Lydia's Fit 'n' Fun team I now work with a vast group of presenters. All have different body shapes and sizes. It's great working with reality people. I am feeling content with myself. I now know what is reality for me.

Mandy Robinson: working mother

Three years ago I weighed nineteen stone. I was a mum with five young children, all of whom had to be born by caesarean. Each time I was pregnant the weight just piled on. A friend and I decided to go along to the *Sunday Mirror* Fit'n'Fun weekend. I had never exercised before, yet I wanted to for the fun. I did not care about my size – the event is for everyone.

The first time I went to Lydia's Legs Bums 'n' Tums class, I stood there looking at the hundreds of people on the floor, all shapes, sizes and ages, all in nice leotards, all except me. I felt so fat, I felt awful. I could hardly do the exercises I was so fat.

I enjoyed the weekend, it was fun being with the

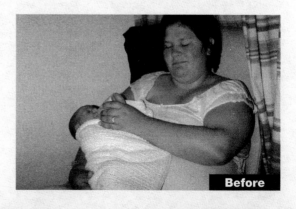

Before

girls but I came home and cried. I hated myself, I wanted to be like all those other people. I had always accepted the fact that I was fat, what else could I expect to be like, after having five caesareans?

After that weekend, I knew I could not stay the way I was, I decided I just had to lose weight. A friend went with me to Boots where I weighed myself, I was nineteen stone. I finally faced the fact that I had to lose it.

I did not want to go to a slimming club, I knew what I had to do. Slimming clubs were too expensive. Instead I kept a food diary and monitored everything I ate. Within the first week I lost one stone. I knew this was only water weight but there was no looking back.

I bought one of Lydia's videos and exercised everyday in front of the telly. My husband did not believe I could do it until I lost the first five stone, then he really encouraged me. Within a year I lost ten stone.

I have been back to Fit'n'Fun every year since. It is just an amazing event, being with everyone and doing so many different classes. Legs Bums 'n' Tums is my favourite because I feel my muscles

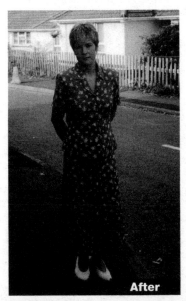

After

working. It is not complicated to follow, it is the mix of aerobic and body conditioning that I need.

Lydia became my inspiration because she is a mum of four and has a realistic build. I have maintained my weight-loss by regular exercise and healthy eating. I still indulge from time to time but I am so conscious of not losing control, I could easily overeat. Now I am a totally different person – I am confident and can do anything now. Although it is funny to say this, I was not miserable when I was fat. Fat people are often happier because they simply do not care anymore.

I have started working now and my weight has dropped to 9st 7lbs. I cannot exercise as often now as I have less time but I will never go back to what I was, especially after I recently had a medical. My doctor cannot believe how healthy I am now because before he was expecting me to be dead within six years if I stayed at nineteen stone. When I was that fat I had no idea my life was in danger.

Elizabeth Macdonald:
mother and recovering anorexic
I have found the ULBT programme the most enjoyable, realistic and achievable work-out programme around. I've always exercised and have an ingrained body-image problem which evolved from being the third daughter in a family of extremely high achievers. I could not cope with family expectations, and from being an athletic teenager I became anorexic from the age of eighteen to twenty-four. I underwent treatment for six years. In those days having a distorted body image was not connected to eating disorders.

During the course of treatment I had, I was given bed rest and daily weighing to achieve a target weight which was monitored on a wall-mounted chart by my bedside. I was also sedated to increase my appetite and reduce my energy levels. My weight fluctuated from 6–9st at 5ft 6". I was not released from medical care until I stabilized my weight at nine stone for six months. I think the treatment I had was good and necessary but nobody helped me deal with the cause of my anorexia. Poor body-image was never discussed. I have had to cope with this myself.

In time, I married and I had three lovely children but I have always had an inner battle with my weight. Everyone seems to be weight obsessed, from girlfriends to doctors.

It was not until I started Lydia's programme that I realised that I could change my perception of weight. Through her programme, I now know that muscle weighs more than fat. I went down a dress size, found my waist again and firmed up. I am not weight-obsessed anymore. Lydia's reality is an inspiration. I have recently had my third child. I exercised throughout my pregnancy under the guidance of Lydia. Two weeks after the birth, I was back into my jeans. I feel fitter and stronger. My recovery from the birth has been so much faster, and, yes, I am coming to terms with my own personal body battle.

Anne Watkins: fifty-three years old

'Go for it': that's my advice to anyone contemplating Lydia's ULBT programme. I am fitter and healthier, have lost weight and gained muscle tone, am now a better skier and tennis player and my posture has changed. It was the ULBT class that sorted me out after I stopped smoking, when I was piling on the weight.

Dawn Thomas: Fit 'n' Fun presenter

I went to Lydia's ULBT programme to tone up my lower body, especially my abdominals. I did the exercise programme three times a week for three months. I lost inches from my hips and toned-up my ~lso gained confidence and I feel almost

time fun and understanding. Soon I was completely hooked. I started to go to other classes. One day I approached Lydia after class to tell her what I thought. She said I had good style and form, and would I consider training to teach. That was it.

Those words of encouragement changed my life. I became a qualified aerobics instructor. Lydia gave me a few classes and I have not looked back since. I have now been teaching for three years. I love it. I would like to say a big thank you to Lydia for changing my life. I hope I will always be able to give my students the same reality message and the understanding that fitness is a lifelong fun commitment.

Alexis Powell: mother of three, forty-four years old

ULBT is a great programme because it really targets all those trouble spots and includes aerobics for fat burning. Using the video I lost a stone and have maintained the weight-loss over the years. I am now more active than ever. I cycle every day and do a work-out three times a week. Lydia's motivated me to maintain a healthier lifestyle. She is the most inspirational fitness presenter I have ever seen.

...hed me through the exercises.
...r technique, while at the same

Fit kit clothing

	Small	Medium	Large	Price
Long-sleeved backless leotard	▧	▧	▧	£24.50
Laced back unitard bike length	▧	▧	▧	£29.95
Front-cross bra top in black or grey (specify colour required)	▧	▧	▧	£14.99
Matching work-out skirt with built-in pants	▧	▧	▧	£24.50
Harem lycra work-out pants	▧	▧	▧	£24.50
Matching lycra long-sleeved top	▧	▧	▧	£14.99
Postage and packing (per item)				£2.95

To order call **0181 741 0215** with your credit card details,
or send a cheque payable to '**Fitcamp Ltd**'
to the address below. Please indicate sizes required.

If you want to go on Lydia's event mailing list or for information on Fit Camps,
please phone 0181 741 0215 or send Freepost to:
Centre for Fitness
41 Overstone Road
Hammersmith
London W6 0AD
Watch out for the Ultimate Legs Bums 'N' Tums video to be released in 1997.

USEFUL ADDRESSES:

For further information:

Aerobic and Fitness Association of America
AFAA Suite 310
15250 Ventura Blvd
Sherman Oaks
California 91403
USA

Association for the Obese
Mrs C Hawkins
20 Brook Meadow Close
Woodford Green
Essex IG8 9NR

Eating Disorders Association
Sackville Place
44 Magdalen Street
Norwich
Norfolk NR3 1JE

Exercise Association
Unit 1 Angel Gate
326 City Road
London EC1 2PT

Fitcamps Ltd
41 Overstone Road
Hammersmith
London W6 0AD

Forza Fitness Equipment
4th Floor
Europe House
World Trade Centre
London E1 9AA

IDEA - The Association for Fitness Professionals
Suite 204
6190 Corner Stone
Court East, San Diego
California 92121
USA

The National Exercise For Life Institute
P.O. Box 2000
Excelsior
MN 55331 - 9967
USA

Recommend further reading on Nutrition:
Anita Bean, The Complete Guide to Sport Nutrition, A + C Black 1994
Beechy Colclough, It is not what you eat, it is why you eat it, Vermilion 1995
Judy Ridgway, Food for Sport, Boxtree 1994

Credits

Thank you to the following companies for kindly supplying shoes, clothing and equipment:
FitCamp: (0181) 748 7483
Nike (UK) Ltd: (0191) 401 6453
Adrian Godden of Energique for designing all my clothing over the years and helping to create my own clothing range: (01376) 551 005
The Leotard Company: (01604) 416 000
Rosie & Company: (0181) 785 9596
Thank you to Forza for supplying equipment for the models.
Thank you to the models:
Kate Jakobsson
Suki Miles
Rayne and Hester Campbell
Illustrations: H. Van De Matten